MANAGING
PMS
NATURALLY

Other books by M. Sara Rosenthal

The Thyroid Sourcebook (4th edition, 2000)

The Gynecological Sourcebook (3rd edition, 1999)

The Pregnancy Sourcebook (3rd edition, 1999)

The Fertility Sourcebook (3rd edition, 1999)

The Breastfeeding Sourcebook (2nd edition, 1998)

The Breast Sourcebook (2nd edition, 1999)

The Gastrointestinal Sourcebook (1997; 1998)

The Type 2 Diabetic Woman (U.S. only; 1999)

The Thyroid Sourcebook for Women (1999)

Women and Sadness (Canada only; 2000)

Women and Depression (U.S. only; 2000)

Women of the '60s Turning 50 (Canada only; 2000)

Women and Passion (Canada only; 2000)

The Canadian Type 2 Diabetes Sourcebook (Canada only; 2002)

50 Ways Series

50 Ways To Prevent Colon Cancer (2000)

50 Ways Women Can Prevent Heart Disease (2000)

50 Ways To Manage Ulcer, Heartburn and Reflux (2001)

50 Ways To Manage Type 2 Diabetes (U.S. only; 2001)

50 Ways To Prevent and Manage Stress (2001)

50 Ways To Fight Depression Without Drugs (2001)

SarahealthGuides

SarahealthGuides are available only at online bookstores such as amazon.com.

Visit **sarahealth.com** for upcoming titles.

Stopping Cancer at the Source (2001)

Women and Unwanted Hair (2001)

MANAGING PMS NATURALLY

A SOURCEBOOK OF

NATURAL SOLUTIONS

M. SARA ROSENTHAL

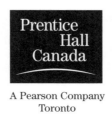

Prentice
Hall
Canada

A Pearson Company
Toronto

Canadian Cataloguing in Publication Data
Rosenthal, M. Sara
    Managing PMS : A sourcebook of natural solutions

ISBN 0-13-065978-9

1. Premenstrual syndrome—Alternative treatment. 2. Premenstrual syndrome—Popular works. 3. Self-care, Health.
4. Naturopathy. I. Title.

RG165.R67 2001   618.1'72   C2001-901241-1

ISBN 0-13-065978-9

Editorial Director, Trade Division: Andrea Crozier
Acquisitions Editor: Nicole de Montbrun
Managing Editor: Tracy Bordian
Copy Editor: Lisa Berland
Proofreader: Dawn Hunter
Cover Design: Mary Opper
Interior Design: Amy Harnden/Mary Opper
Cover Image: Steve Taylor/Stone
Author Photograph: Greg Edwards
Production Manager: Kathrine Pummell
Page Layout: Gail Ferreira Ng-A-Kien

This publication contains the opinions and ideas of its author and is designed to provide useful advice in regard to the subject matter covered. The herbs and other treatments in this book are described for the information and education of readers. They are not a replacement for diagnosis and treatment by qualified health professionals. The author and publisher are not engaged in rendering health or other professional services in this publication. This publication is not intended to provide a basis for action in particular circumstances without consideration by a competent professional. The author and publisher expressly disclaim any responsibility for any liability, loss, or risk, personal or otherwise, which is incurred as a consequence, directly or indirectly, of the use and application of any of the contents of this book. To obtain recommendations appropriate to your particular situation, please consult a qualified health care provider. The herbal information in this book is provided for education purposes only and is not meant to be used without consulting a qualified health practitioner who is trained in herbal medicine.

ATTENTION: CORPORATIONS
Books are available at quantity discounts with bulk purchase for educational, business, or sales promotional use. For information, please email or write to: Pearson PTR Canada, Special Sales, PTR Division, 26 Prince Andrew Place, Don Mills, Ontario, M3C 2T8. Email ss.corp@pearsoned.com. Please supply: title of book, ISBN, quantity, how the book will be used, date needed.

Visit the Pearson PTR Canada Web site! Send us your comments, browse our catalogues, and more.
www.pearsonptr.ca

1 2 3 4 5   WEB   05 04 03 02 01

Printed and bound in Canada.

A Pearson Company

Contents

Detailed Contents

Acknowledgments

I wish to thank the following people, whose expertise and dedication helped to lay so much of the groundwork for this book (listed alphabetically): Gillian Arsenault, M.D., C.C.F.P., I.B.L.C., F.R.C.P.; Pamela Craig, M.D., F.A.C.S., Ph.D.; Masood Kahthamee, M.D., F.A.C.O.G.; Debra Lander, M.D., F.R.C.P.; Gary May, M.D., F.R.C.P.; James McSherry, M.B., Ch.B., F.C.F.P., F.R.C.G.P., F.A.A.F.P., F.A.B.M.P.; Suzanne Pratt, M.D., FA.C.O.G.; Wm Warren Rudd, M.D., F.R.C.S., F.A.C.S., Colon and Rectal Surgeon and Founder and Director of The Rudd Clinic For Diseases of the Colon and Rectum (Toronto); and Robert Volpe, M.D., F.R.C.P., F.A.C.P.

William Harvey, Ph.D., L.L.B., University of Toronto Joint Centre for Bioethics, whose devotion to bioethics has inspired me, continues to support my work and makes it possible for me to have the courage to question and challenge issues in health care and medical ethics. Irving Rootman, Ph.D., Director, University of Toronto Centre for Health Promotion, continues to encourage my interest in primary prevention and health promotion issues. Helen Lenskyj, Ph.D., Professor, Department of Sociology and Equity Studies, Ontario Institute for Studies in Education/University of Toronto, and Laura M. Purdy, Ph.D., Department of Philosophy, University of Toronto, and Bioethicist, University of Toronto, Joint Centre for Bioethics, have been central figures in my understanding the complexities of women's health issues and feminist bioethics.

Larissa Kostoff, my editorial consultant, worked very hard to bring this book into being. And finally, Nicole de Montbrun, my editor, championed this project and saw how important it was for all these health issues to come together for this unique women's health concern.

Introduction: It's Okay to Feel Like a Natural Woman

The most important piece of information you can get from this book is this: Menstruation, and all of the bodily changes that occur before, during, and after, are *normal*. The term "PMS" is more commonly known as "premenstrual syndrome" (in the United Kingdom it is also known as "premenstrual tension," or PMT). For the purposes of this book, I am renaming PMS **premenstrual signs**. I dislike the terms "syndrome" and "symptoms" because they imply a diseased state. Now, when I refer to premenstrual signs, I am referring to the many physical discomforts and shifts in moods and emotional responses women experience during this time due to the normal fluctuations of hormones. These fluctuations happen to us during pregnancy, breast-feeding, menopause, and throughout our life cycle as we age. We are human women on the planet Earth who experience our hormones. This is normal and natural and not a disease.

We are also living in a world that was not built for us: our economy and the buildings we work in, for example, were designed for males — not bodies that menstruate, get pregnant, breast-feed, and go through menopause. As well, unfair power arrangements in both our working and intimate relationships predispose women to depression. So it's important to recognize that there are more things going on before and during our periods than simply our periods; there are *social causes* for mood swings, and *social causes* that exacerbate the normal physical discomforts that we go through during the various stages of our lives. In other words, your premenstrual signs may be aggravated by the conditions of your life, which I will delve into more in Chapters 2, 3, and 4.

That said, as I write this introduction, television ads are currently telling roughly 90 percent of all menstruating women that they may indeed have a disease known as *premenstrual dysphoric disorder (PDD)*. This term simply means "unhappy before your period." The television ads suggest you speak to your doctor about going on Sarafem, which is a new name for an old drug: Prozac. Eli Lilly, the makers of Prozac, have lost their patent for fluoxetine hydrochloride (the generic drug name for Prozac) and are trying to carve out a new market. Selling its popular antidepressant to 90 percent of menstruating women sounds like a great way to recapture market share to me. The only problem is this: How can 90 percent of menstruating women have a disease? And if you believe this is a reasonable question to ask, then you are a woman who can greatly benefit from this book.

Virtually all women in their childbearing years have premenstrual signs; Chapters 3 and 4 discuss all of the physical and emotional changes in great detail. As we age, our premenstrual signs can become more severe, especially as we approach our peri-menopause (a term that means "around menopause"), which is usually somewhere in our mid-to-late 40s. Premenstrual signs occur roughly 14 days before your period and disappear when your get your period, or just after. The main question is: *Should* premenstrual signs be treated? And is it right to think of these signs as a "disease" or disorder, medicating them with antidepressants, tranquilizers, water pills, or synthetically produced hormones? Even if you are the one who wants your doctor to prescribe medication for your premenstrual changes, you should still consider this question.

Traditionally, women's complaints about premenstrual signs have been viewed as either psychological or written off as part of the biological lot of women. Many women have difficulty admitting they suffer from premenstrual signs for fear of compromising their position in the workplace. But virtually all women experience some premenstrual signs. It's how *you* experience these signs, and how severely they affect *you*, that determine whether these premenstrual signs warrant remedying through natural means, or, in the extreme, through medical interventions, such as harsh medications or synthetic hormones.

Ninety percent of women who menstruate experience premenstrual signs of some sort. Of this group, half will experience the more traditional premenstrual signs, such as breast tenderness, bloating, food cravings, irritability, and mood swings. Many women perceive these signs as indications that their bodies are "in tune" or "on schedule" and that all is well. In other words, the signs are natural markers of a healthy menstrual cycle. If you fall into this group, you may find that moderately adjusting your diet or adding one or two of the dietary or herbal supplements discussed in this book can dramatically reduce your premenstrual discomforts.

Thirty-five to 40 percent of menstruating women experience the same signs as the first group, but in a more severe form. In other words, they have *really* tender breasts, so sensitive that they hurt if someone just lightly touches them; severe bloating, to the extent that they gain about five pounds before their periods; instead of just food cravings, they may suddenly find that they have voracious appetites; instead of just being irritable, they may find that they become impossible to be around; and so on. Even these more severe signs are considered to be normal experiences. If you fall into this group, you may find that more rigorous dietary adjustments and supplements, in combination with herbal remedies and physical activity, can dramatically reduce your level of discomfort. You may also benefit from ruling out other causes for your discomforts and may even want to explore natural progesterone supplements.

Roughly 3 to 10 percent of menstruating women (the latest statistics hover around 3 to 4 percent) suffer from incapacitating discomforts that affect their ability to function. These women experience discomforts that interfere with their quality of life, such as profound mood swings; sudden, unexplainable sadness; irritability; sudden or unexplainable anger; feelings of anxiety or being "on edge;" depression; hopelessness; self-deprecating thoughts; and the range of physical discomforts discussed in Chapter 4, such as tender breasts, bloating, and so on. In the psychiatric literature, even women with hysterectomies and oophorectomies (removal of their ovaries) were found to experience these symptoms. It is considered sound and good medicine to offer this group of women antidepressants as a treatment for their PMS, even though incapacitating discomforts can still be managed through natural remedies.

If you fall into this group, it's important to first rule out other causes for your physical and emotional discomforts, such as stress or an underlying depression that has social causes and has more to do with your life's conditions; or you may have reactions to other synthetic hormones or medications you are taking that get aggravated by fluctuating hormones around the time of your period. Next, take a long hard look at your diet and activity patterns. Adjusting your diet, adding supplements and herbs, and becoming more active can really make a difference. Finally, you may benefit from natural progesterone supplements, which I discuss in Chapter 8. I urge you to consider synthetic hormones, antidepressants, anti-anxiety agents, and other medications as a last resort. These are strong medications that carry a long list of side effects.

This book is designed to help you *help yourself.* Use the information in the book to ease your premenstrual discomforts and, at the same time, your discomfort with taking harsh medicine when more reasonable and safer alternatives exist.

PMS IS NOT A DISEASE

Menstruation is a powerful force of nature that has affected human culture for centuries. But a force of nature is not the same thing as a disease. PMS is short for *premenstrual signs,* as I explain in the introduction. It is the power of PMS, and the way they can transform our emotional responses, that were the target of witch hunters in the Middle Ages and psychiatric labeling in the 20th century. For example, studies have shown that women can be so much more aggressive before their periods that women in prison were studied and found to be more likely to have committed crimes while under the influence of PMS. One study that looked at autopsies of women who committed suicide found that 20 out of 23 of the women were in their premenstrual phase at the time. Of course, these studies did not consider so many other variables (such as the backgrounds of the women and the social causes for their crimes or suicides) that many of these PMS statistics are meaningless. Catching women 14 days prior to their periods takes a pretty wide net; chances are, at least half of the women you find at random on the street will be premenstrual. But the fact that these studies were published at all reveals how much PMS is still feared in our culture.

Cultural Attitudes

A World Health Organization study on cultural attitudes to PMS revealed that women's bodily changes are influenced by cultural perceptions. Women are more likely to feel sick instead of "normal for this time of the month" because PMS has been labeled a disease, syndrome, or disorder.

The premenstrual mood changes women experience, such as anger, aggression, or "feeling out of control," are considered perfectly normal emotional responses for men, who frequently display rage and aggression. Perhaps the mood changes are nature's way of ensuring women express their feelings. Tears, for example, contain high levels of stress hormones, which, we know from other research, block the action of progesterone receptors, which are the "root system" that carries the hormone progesterone to the various "branches" or body parts. As I suggest in Chapter 3, "The Emotional Premenstrual Signs," perhaps the mood changes are nature's way of ensuring smooth hormonal action! Perhaps expressing our passions and feelings is good for our reproductive health. The problem with expressing emotion is not the emotion but the cultural setting in which we live, which does not allow us to be emotional, passionate beings.

Anthropological studies on menstruating women find, time and time again, that women are considered more powerful around menstruation. Tribal rituals involve isolating women around the time of their periods because of this power, but in some modern cultures, it's become twisted so that women are forced into isolation because they are seen as unclean, as, for example, in the Jewish religion.

The Power of Our Blood

A very real power women possess is the power to attract/repel animals or manipulate plants with the scent of their menstrual blood. In hunting cultures, women were adept at using menstrual blood for tracking, tricking, and trapping animals. In fact, Shamanism and sorcery grew from this knowledge. In my own experiences, I have witnessed this power, but did not understand it until much later.

While traveling alone in the Middle East in my early 20s, I came across a stray German shepherd who was very large. I am afraid of dogs, especially German shepherds. But this dog began to follow me all through one small town — faithfully. When I stopped, he stopped; when I turned, he turned. I was amused, but somewhat worried. I tried to lose the dog by going into a large hotel on the town's tourist strip. I went through a rotating door and left the dog outside the hotel as I made my way into an elevator and to a fancy bar. I sat down and ordered a drink. Ten minutes later, the dog found me and lay down by my feet. The hotel manager asked me to get rid of the dog or leave the hotel. I insisted that the dog was not mine and got up. The dog got up, too. I sat down, and the dog lay down. The hotel manager laughed and called me a liar; he told me to leave the premises with "my dog." The dog was gone from outside my hostel in the morning, but for many days I wondered what had attracted it to me. Then it occurred to me: I was having my period at the time. It was my menstrual blood that attracted the dog. In hindsight, I now realize that as a woman traveling alone in a strange country, I could have benefited from a guard dog. I had unwittingly attracted a guard dog, which responded to me as though he were sent to an expensive dog training school, with the sheer power of my menstrual blood.

Several myths also revolve around the "transformative" powers of menstrual blood. Some ancient cultures believed that the embryo was made from menstrual blood, which outwardly made sense because we do not menstruate during pregnancy. Other ancient cultures compared menstruation to flowering plants and fruits. As the flower opens its red petals, it forms fruit, just as women do.

Corn is often associated with the menstrual cycle myths in horticultural societies, which depend on females. This can be seen in a Cherokee myth called "River, Blood, and Corn." The story involves a Cherokee matriarch whose menstrual blood turns into a wild boy (a symbol of the aggression and power women display before menstruation).

The wild boy then catches her in the act of making a meal of seven ears of corn (perhaps representing the seven days before menstruation) and beans for her family, using her body. The ears of corn fall from her vaginal opening, and the beans come out of her nipples. The wild boy calls her a sorceress, and the matriarch says: "You have seen me and now I must die; it's time for my transformation."

From Shamanism to Shameful

Menstruation went from a positive, powerful force of nature to a shameful experience that women had to conceal. Eve Ensler clearly shows us the "shame" in her chapter on menstruation, entitled "I Was 12. And My Mother Slapped Me." Ensler writes:

> I interviewed many women about menstruation. There was a choral thing that began to occur, a kind of wild collective song. Women echoed each other. I let the voices bleed into one another. I got lost in the bleeding. (Ensler, Eve, *The Vagina Monologues*, 33)

One of the echoes we hear in Ensler's chapter includes images like the following: "I was so afraid. I started putting the used pads in brown paper bags in the dark storage places under the roof" (Ensler, 34).

Karen Houppert tackles the politics of concealing menstruation in her book *The Curse, Confronting the Last Unmentionable Taboo: Menstruation*:

> Research on American's attitudes toward menstruation is very hard to come by. Periods are not a popular dissertation topic. Prestige and altruism rarely drive scientists to seek new cures for cramps. The U.S. government, which has only recently recognized the importance of studying women's health issues by creating the National Institute of Health's Office of Women's Health, mostly limits its analysis of menstruation to one question: Does it render women unfit for combat? ... When the experts do focus their attention on menstruation, it's to emphasize pathology: premenstrual syndrome. While studies on healthy women are hard to come by, studies on angry, depressed, and unreasonable women fill the pages of professional journals. (Houppert, Karen, *The Curse, Confronting the Last Unmentionable Taboo: Menstruation*, 5)

How PMS Became a Disease

Why are you led to believe that PMS constitute a disease that needs to be treated? The answer is simple: You live in a Western culture where *everything* is medicalized and pathologized — from womb to tomb. It's not just PMS that are medicalized. This trend can be seen with care for menopause, pregnancy and prenatal care, pediatric care (for example, many children are being "diagnosed" with "behavior disorders" who in the past were considered normal), psychological care (for example, people are put on medication for angst, anxiety, and depression that have social causes), and so on. In short, *all* the normal physical processes of the human body have been "pathologized" by medicine.

Most frequently, it is women's normal physical processes that are subject to the mass marketing of prevention drugs or untested therapies. For example, in our 20s and 30s, we are sold drugs to prevent pregnancy and "regulate" our cycles. In our 30s and 40s (and now 50s), we are put on fertility drugs to "regulate" our cycles so we *can* get pregnant. And in our 50s and beyond, we are put on estrogen replacement drugs to "regulate" our cycles, too, and to prevent health problems associated with estrogen loss. There are many other health conditions for which questionable drugs are sold to women, such as obesity (fen/phen) and breast cancer (tamoxifen).

The "Syndrome" Label

PMS was first labeled "premenstrual syndrome" in 1953 by a British physician, Dr. Katharina Dalton, whom I will refer to throughout this book. Dalton began treating premenstrual discomforts as early as 1948; she was working during a time when virtually no women were doctors, and when most women were dismissed by male doctors as "crazy" when they reported premenstrual complaints. It was Dalton who validated women's premenstrual discomforts and mood changes by recognizing a group of symptoms that were universal to premenstrual women. She was the first to carefully itemize a set of symptoms and label them a syndrome. Dalton's definition, which is still used today, is that PMS means "the recurrence of symptoms *before* menstruation with *complete absence* of symptoms *after* menstruation" (Dalton, 1999, 7). The symptoms comprise all the premenstrual mood changes I discuss in Chapter 3, "The Emotional Premenstrual Signs," as well as the premenstrual physical discomforts discussed in Chapter 4, "The Physical Premenstrual Signs."

Dalton's first book, *The Premenstrual Syndrome,* was published in 1964. She added *The Menstrual Cycle* in 1969. She is most famous for her pioneering work in treating PMS with progesterone therapy, and her book *Once A Month: Understanding and Treating PMS*, first published in 1978, is in its sixth edition and still going strong.

Critics of Dalton, such as Karen Houppert, author of *The Curse*, insist that Dalton's work ought to be challenged because the criteria she outlines for PMS are nearly

50 years old. They have become an industry standard, commonly treated with "mega-doses of the hormone progesterone" (Houppert, 146). I discuss progesterone therapy in Chapter 8, "Natural Progesterone Therapy for PMS." Dalton has to be viewed, however, as a true pioneer in a field nobody was interested in studying. And to her credit, her many years of PMS research have laid the groundwork for the natural approaches used to remedy premenstrual discomforts. Dalton's research revealed two core findings: that blood sugar and stress affect PMS. Today, naturopaths and other practitioners of alternative approaches to PMS all acknowledge the role of diet and stress in controlling the severity of PMS. Dalton was also careful to distinguish the difference between premenstrual depression and depression in the absence of PMS. It is her criteria that were used to describe PMS-related depression in the *Diagnostic and Statistical Manual of Mental Disorders*, Fourth Edition (DSM-IV), which is the bible of diagnostic criteria for the psychiatric community.

Dalton's negative contribution to the study of PMS is her belief that women are not responsible for their actions due to PMS-related mood swings. She has appeared as a witness in court many times for women who commit crimes during PMS, and she lists several questionable statistics in her books relating crime and PMS. Dalton has no problem blaming PMS for the range of women's social problems, including bad marriages, violent behavior, and eating disorders.

Subclassifications

PMS experts who followed Dalton further classified PMS, making it even more technical:

- **PMS-A.** The *A* is for anxiety, and women with PMS-A are said to suffer from premenstrual anxiety, irritability, and emotional instability related to too much estrogen and not enough progesterone.

- **PMS-C.** The *C* is for cravings, and women with PMS-C are said to experience increased appetite, cravings for sweets, headaches, fatigue, fainting spells, and heart palpitations. These, by the way, are all signs of unstable blood sugar, which leads to progesterone deficiency. (See Chapter 4, "The Physical Premenstrual Signs.")

- **PMS-D.** The *D* is for depression. Women with PMS-D are said to suffer from decreased levels of estrogen premenstrually, which cause changes in serotonin levels. The depression will disappear when the period starts.

- **PMS-H.** The *H* is for hyperhydration, which means bloating. (It would make more sense to label it PMS-B, which would neatly fit between PMS-A and PMS-C!)

Women with PMS-H are said to suffer from water retention symptoms, such as bloating, breast tenderness, congestion, and swollen hands and feet due to an excess of androgen levels, which could be stress-related.

The "Dysphoric Disorder" Label

It was "PMS-D" and "PMS-A" that caught the attention of the psychiatric community. In 1983, the National Institute of Mental Health established diagnostic guidelines for PMS for mental health professionals who were trying to help women with premenstrual mood swings. By 1987, PMS was renamed *late luteal phase dysphoric disorder*, which meant "women unhappy with their periods during the last phase of the menstrual cycle." It was then changed in 1994 to a catchier label: *premenstrual dysphoric disorder (PDD),* or "unhappy before your period" and was included in the *Diagnostic and Statistical Manual of Mental Disorders, Fourth Edition* (DSM-IV), under the subheading "Mood Disorders Not Otherwise Specified." Until 1973, homosexuality was labeled a disorder in the DSM, too.

The psychiatric labeling of premenstrual changes as a mental disorder poses more problems than Dalton's labeling of PMS because it labels the premenstrual woman "crazy." Sharon Golub, in her 1992 book *Periods,* questions why changes in mood have to be a problem: "Rather than accepting the cyclic changes as the norm, some baseline from which we are not expected to deviate becomes the norm" (Houppert, 169). Psychologist Paula Caplan, author of *They Say You're Crazy* and an outspoken critic of the psychiatric labeling of PMS/PDD told the *Washington Post:* "The APA says, 'We'll believe what you women tell us about how you're feeling—but you've got to let us call you mentally ill'" (Houppert, 184–5).

The DSM-IV makes it clear that the emotional changes women experience prior to their period (depression, anxiety, and irritability) are the major features of PDD, not the physical signs of breast tenderness, bloating, and weight gain. Yet the ads for Sarafem (an antidepressant commonly prescribed for PDD) show one woman arguing with her husband and another frustrated because she can't button her pants. The DSM-IV stipulates that to be labeled with PDD, the emotional changes have to be severe enough to disrupt a woman's ability to function, and must present before the period begins, disappearing after the period ends.

Says Houppert:

> Originally confined to medical texts, PMS has slipped so comfortably into our cultural lexicon today that it explains away a colleague's crankiness, a couple's marital strife, or a mother's short-tempered treatment of her kids.... More troubling, though, is the way in which the term has become a convenient catchall for women's

complaints, a way of discounting women's anger—and their often legitimate concerns—by attributing their dissatisfaction to hormones. (Conversely, it provides an acceptable excuse for women who are reluctant to claim their anger: "I was not myself.") Because a woman's anger affects others—husbands, colleagues, family—society has been quick to embrace PMS as an explanation for it. And anxious to cure it. (Houppert, 141)

This acceptance of the approach to PMS may explain why many women actually ask for an antidepressant as a treatment for their PMS. If the culture tells them enough times that they are "sick," they begin to behave that way, and believe it themselves.

A Blast from the Past

This isn't the first time in which doctors have manufactured a mental illness around female biology and behaviors. The most profound example of how psychiatry and women's social history are intertwined is the diagnosis and treatment of "hysteria," a term that remained in the vernacular of medicine from the fourth century B.C. until 1952, when the American Psychiatric Association finally stopped using it. Hysteria was listed as the most common women's disease next to fevers, and it was thought to be a disease caused by sexual dissatisfaction (or longing) commonly diagnosed in virgins, young widows, and nuns, who were discouraged from the terrible sin of masturbation. Marriage was considered a cure, but clearly, it failed to cure many women. Hysteria was also thought to plague women with more passionate natures.

In their 1978 book *For Her Own Good*, Barbara Ehrenreich and Dierdre English describe an "ovary illness" that was thought in the 19th century to be responsible for personality problems in women. It was believed, in fact, that the ovaries controlled the personality. Oophorectomy (a.k.a. ovariectomy) was the cure, then called "ovariotomies." The ovary illness coincided with the Suffragette Movement, sometimes called the First Wave of Feminism.

In her 1972 book, *Women and Madness*, Phyllis Chesler exposed the deeply embedded sexism of the system that had been mistreating and incarcerating women for centuries. She also exposed the so-called "symptoms" of depression and hysteria as simply *healthy* responses to a sick role women were playing in society. Chesler dared to say: yes, oppression is *depressing*! When the women's movement re-emerged in the late 1960s and early 1970s (in academic circles this is known as "post-modernist" or "second wave" feminism, to distinguish it from the first wave, which took place at the beginning of the 20th century), it liberated women from many of their so-called mental illnesses.

The Drugging of Premenstrual Women

In 1995, an article in the *New England Journal of Medicine* announced good results in using Prozac for PMS/PDD. The study was conducted in Canada and funded by Eli Lilly, the makers of Prozac. It involved 700 Canadian women dispersed throughout seven different clinics. The study announced a 50 to 75 percent improvement in PMS symptoms for women who took Prozac daily. Although Prozac had been widely prescribed to women anyway for "garden variety" depressions by general practitioners and gynecologists, there was now solid evidence that Prozac could be used for PMS. The medical logic for putting a woman who suffers from temporary depression that passes in a few days on a daily antidepressant is the belief that women who have PDD are more at risk for developing major depression. But taking an antidepressant and stopping it abruptly can create a much worse depression. So what the "major depression" doctors see when women try to get off the antidepressant may be *iatrogenic* depression, meaning a depression caused directly by the medical treatment itself.

It has been considered standard medical practice to put women who fall into the PDD criteria on antidepressants. Seventy-five percent of all antidepressants are prescribed to women; in 2000, more than 13 million individual antidepressant prescriptions were filled in Canada alone. Women are frequently told that their PDD will worsen with time, and the antidepressant will prevent an underlying "mood disorder" from developing. I'm no math whiz, but there's something wrong when PDD officially affects only 3 to 4 percent of the general female population, but the dispensing of antidepressants to women increased tremendously after 1995, to the point where two-thirds of antidepressant users are women. Eighty percent of the new Prozac prescriptions written for women were written by doctors other than psychiatrists; it stands to reason that many of these prescriptions were PMS-based.

Forty percent of women taking antidepressants feel sicker from the side effects of the drug than they did before they went on it. It is a fact that antidepressants work for only about 60 percent of the users. For more information on antidepressants, see Chapter 9, "Prescription Drugs Used for PMS."

Managing PMS "naturally" cannot happen until you understand what's wrong with the current thinking about PMS, and with some of the *unnatural* therapies and medications that are used to suppress what is normal female biology. As I state in the introduction, our current society was not designed to accommodate the biology of women — bodies that menstruate, get pregnant, breast-feed, and go through menopause. That said, our bodies were not designed to go through the stresses our current society imposes. We see the effects of stress in a number of ways, but it is our hormonal cycle — the "lifeblood" that defines our gender and sex, moods, and emotions so much of the time — that can be altered. Arming ourselves with the right information can help to offset the outside interference that affects our normal biology. And we can do it naturally, without unnatural substances that can interfere with our bodies even more.

2

CYCLE-LOGICAL MATTERS

Managing your premenstrual signs and reducing some of the discomforts depend on knowing your cycle. This chapter serves as a refresher course on the menstrual cycle, explaining some of the common menstrual cycle problems women have and ways to remedy them. It also discusses all of the safety and environmental issues surrounding menstrual products under the section "What to Wear For Your Period."

The first period, clinically known as *menarche,* is probably one of the most powerful psychological, sociological, and physiological occurrences in any woman's life. It is her rite of passage. Once we begin our menstrual cycle, we enter into a completely different physiological phase: our reproductive years.

Even today, many young women don't understand what the menstrual cycle is; they feel shame, fear, anxiety, and depression about their first periods, and as a result, have very negative experiences. Sometimes the negative first experience has to do with painful periods and cramping (discussed later in this chapter), but often the negative experience is linked to false information about what a period actually is, and what it means. The negativity of menstruation is then reinforced when we become sexually active. For example, many men are repulsed by the menstrual flow and refrain from petting or having intercourse with menstruating women.

There is also a negative mythology about menstruation, which traces all the way back to the book of Genesis. The term "the curse," for example, comes from the story of Adam and Eve. In a nutshell, the story goes that Eve's punishment for biting the apple — the forbidden fruit from the Tree of Knowledge — was to be cursed with painful childbirth ever after. The biblical and completely erroneous interpretation is that the period is a monthly reminder to women that it is *they* who kicked man out of paradise (something men keep reminding women about, even though it is more accurate to say *humanity* was kicked out of Eden).

Unfortunately, the negative mythology and imagery associated with menstruation has been created by our patriarchal culture. Until this century, very little was understood about the menstrual cycle, and nothing was known about hormones. Menstruation was thus seen as a mysterious enigma, and the emotional signs leading up to menstruation were feared, branded as a kind of hysteria by the male medical profession. Since women have been living in a patriarchal society for so many centuries, they, too, have become quasi-believers in the "evils" of menstruation, believing that medicating and masking our cycles is appropriate.

The Moon Cycle

A normal menstrual cycle is more accurately a moon cycle. Interestingly, the only event in human life that corresponds to the lunar calendar is menstruation. Time itself was probably first measured by the moon's phases. One of the problems with the current Western calendar is that the months don't coincide exactly with the solar year. In our system, the months have been made to fit by Gregory XIII (which is why it's called the Gregorian calendar), who gave them an arbitrary number of days unrelated to the moon calendar. So our calendar actually puts us *out* of synch with the moon.

The word *menstrual* comes from the Latin word *mens* meaning "month"; the word *month* comes from the root word "moon." The Greek word for "moon" is *mene*, so *menstruation* actually means "moon change." (In some dictionaries, the root word for "month" and "menstruation" is "measure.")

Countless other languages and cultures link menstruation to the moon as well. German peasants literally refer to menstruation as "the moon," while the French term for menstruation is *le moment de la lune* ("the moment of the moon"). Mandingos, Susus, and Kongos also call menstruation "the moon," while in parts of East Africa, menstruation is thought to be *caused* by the new moon. The Papuans believe that the moon has intercourse with girls, triggering their periods; the Maori call menstruation "moon sickness"; the Fueginas call the moon "The Lord of the Women." Clearly the belief that the lunar cycle is identical to the menstrual cycle is universal.

Some remarkable physical evidence connects the moon to menstruation even more. For example, the cervix, *metra* in Greek (referring again to the word measurement; also called the "meter of a woman") changes color, size, and position during menstruation. In fact, when it's viewed using a speculum (an instrument doctors use to open up the vagina), the cervix has been said to resemble a globe. Even the embryo is shaped like the moon: It starts out round and full, and as it becomes a fetus, curves like the half-moon.

All this evidence suggests that perhaps women are far more in tune to the natural "rhythms" of the universe than they think. Meanwhile, comprehending the similarities between the menstrual and lunar cycles is crucial for understanding what a healthy, normal menstrual cycle really is. Women are also in tune with other women's cycles; the cycles of two women living together will often synchronize.

What Is "Normal"?

The menstrual cycle is in fact a "hormonal cycle." The menstrual cycle is driven by a symphony of hormones that trigger each other, stopping and starting, flooding and tapering in a regular rhythm each month. Every woman's hormones dance to a different tune — but rarely does the cycle correspond to the Gregorian calendar.

Low levels of sex hormones are continuously produced during a woman's reproductive years. But it is the continuous *fluctuation* of hormones that establishes the menstrual cycle and any premenstrual signs.

The main organs involved in the cycle are the hypothalamus (a part of the brain), the pituitary gland, and the ovaries. The hypothalamus is like the omniscient figure, watching over the cycle and controlling the symphony of hormones from above. It tells the pituitary gland to start the hormonal process, and the pituitary gland in turn signals the ovaries to "do their thing." The hypothalamus is sensitive to the fluctuating levels of hormones produced by the ovaries. When the estrogen drops below a certain level, the hypothalamus turns on *gonadotropin-releasing hormone (GnRH),* which stimulates the pituitary gland to release *follicle-stimulating hormone (FSH).* FSH triggers the growth of 10 to 20 ovarian follicles (small pouches), but only one of them will mature fully; the others will start to degenerate sometime before ovulation. As the follicles grow, they secrete estrogen in increasing amounts. The estrogen affects the lining of the uterus, signaling it to grow, or proliferate (the proliferatory phase). When the egg approaches maturity inside the mature follicle, the follicle secretes a burst of progesterone in addition to the estrogen. This progesterone/estrogen "combo" triggers the hypothalamus to secrete GnRH, which signals the pituitary gland to secrete FSH and *luteinizing hormone (LH).* The FSH/LH levels peak and signal the follicle to release the egg. This is ovulation.

To simplify, imagine a row of dominos standing on end. The hypothalamus, which sends out the GnRH, causes the first domino to fall; the second domino is FSH, which falls and touches the third domino, LH; and so on. When all the dominos have fallen, you menstruate.

Under the influence of LH, the follicle changes its function and is now called a *corpus luteum,* secreting decreasing amounts of estrogen and increasing amounts of progesterone. The progesterone influences the estrogen-primed uterine lining to secrete fluids that nourish the egg (the secretory phase). Immediately after ovulation, FSH returns to a normal or base level, and the LH decreases gradually as the progesterone increases. If the egg is fertilized, the corpus luteum continues to secrete estrogen and progesterone to maintain the pregnancy. In this case, the corpus luteum is stimulated by *human chorionic gonadotropin (HCG),* a hormone that is secreted by the developing placenta. If the egg isn't fertilized, the corpus luteum degenerates until it becomes nonfunctioning; at this point it is called a *corpus albicans*. As the degeneration progresses, the progesterone levels decrease. The decreased progesterone fails to maintain the uterine lining, which causes it to shed. Then, the whole thing starts again.

Most girls have their first period about the middle of puberty, at around 11 or 12 years of age. The first few periods are sporadic, and it's not uncommon for periods to be irregular for a couple of years. Women continue to have periods until about 48 or 49 years of age, and then the periods start to get sporadic again, tapering off as menopause sets in.

Few cycles are absolutely 28 days long. Where does that number come from? It is only an average, representing the cycle length of thousands of women added together and divided by the number of women. It is therefore a *statistical* average, not a figure that refers to the typical number of days in a woman's cycle. Menstrual cycles range anywhere from 20 to 40 days, and the bleeding lasts anywhere from two to eight days, with four to six days being the average.

There's a big difference between your own cycle and a calendar month, however. If you tell your doctor that you get your period on the 15th of every month, for example, you're actually stating the impossible. Since each month has a different number of days, unless you were consistently irregular you couldn't begin menstruating on exactly the 15th of each month.

Finally, it's important to count *the first day of bleeding as day one of your cycle.* Many women count the first day of clear discharge *after* their periods as day one, but this is not as accurate. What's the difference? Since ovulation always takes place roughly 14 days before your period, five days off in your counting could radically interfere with your family planning. Second, if you're on the pill, the first day of bleeding is *always* counted as day one. If you're planning to go on or off the pill, your cycle is more accurately tracked by using the same counting method. Third, doctors always count the first day of bleeding as day one of the cycle.

Many of us assume that our menstrual flow is strictly blood, but this is not so. Menstrual fluid is made from a variety of ingredients: cervical and vaginal mucus, degenerated endometrial particles, and blood. The fluid does not smell until it comes into contact with the bacteria in the air and starts to decompose.

Irregular Cycles: Metrorrhagia

One of the most common gynecological problems is an irregular menstrual cycle. But before you jump to the conclusion that you're irregular, it's important to remember that being regular doesn't mean your cycle is the same number of days each time. One month your cycle may be 29 days, and the next month it may be 31 days. This is still considered regular. It's also normal to be lighter one month and heavier the next. So long as you're menstruating every 20 to 40 days, it's a sign that you're ovulating.

Another common misperception about irregular cycles is the belief that unless you have a period every four weeks (again, the statistical average) you're irregular. This is not true. Some women menstruate every three weeks, which is normal for them; some menstruate every five weeks, which is also normal for them. The only times you should be concerned is if your period consistently yo-yos: three weeks, then four weeks, then five weeks, then three weeks, and so on. When this happens, it's usually a sign that you're not ovulating regularly. This is common in young girls after they first begin menstruating. If your period only jumps around once or twice a year, there isn't anything to worry about. Occasional stress is usually the culprit when this happens.

When You've Skipped a Period

Once in a while, women may skip a period and then experience a heavier flow with their next period. This is extremely common. Women who are trying to get pregnant, however, often fear that this is a miscarriage — so early that it simply feels like a heavy period. This is usually not the case. Although it's *possible* for a pregnancy not to take and for the embryo to expel in the menstrual flow, it's rare and occurs in fewer than 1 percent of women. If this were to occur, it would be so early a pregnancy that the term "miscarriage" would be totally inappropriate; it would simply be a pregnancy that wasn't yet established, technically called a "blighted ovum." Most cases of skipping one period are caused by stress. The flow is heavier after a skipped period because the estrogen has been building up in the endometrium longer, and there is more lining than usual that needs to be shed. In essence, you would have built up two cycles' worth of lining, so the flow is naturally heavier than normal.

It's also common to skip a period altogether and *not* experience a heavier flow the next time around. This means you actually skipped an *ovulation* cycle and did not produce a lining in your endometrium that would support a pregnancy. In this case, there wasn't a lining to shed. It's not unusual to skip one or two periods a year; it is unusual to skip them more often than that, however.

Causes of Irregular or Missed Cycles

The number one cause of irregular or skipped periods is emotional stress, which is discussed more in Chapters 3 and 4. The typical scenario is worrying that you might be pregnant and then actually missing your period *because* you're worried. Other stress-related situations revolve around career changes, job loss, a death in the family, moving, exams, and stressful workloads. It's not really understood why stress can cause you to miss a cycle, but it is considered a protective mechanism, a sort of primal parachute in the female body. The body senses the stress levels and decides somehow to stop ovulation for that month, preventing a "stressed" pregnancy.

Overdieting and overexercising can also affect your cycle. For example, sudden weight loss could cause you to miss your period or cause a long bout of irregular cycles. Overexercising can also cause you to miss your period, and it's actually not unusual for female athletes to stop menstruating when they're in training.

Another possible cause of irregular cycles could be a thyroid disorder of some sort. The thyroid gland regulates your metabolism by secreting thyroid hormone. When the gland is overactive (and secretes too much thyroid hormone), known as *hyperthyroidism*, you can either miss periods or have a much longer cycle than normal. Meanwhile, your period is shorter, with a scanty or light flow. On the flip side, when the gland is underactive (and doesn't secrete *enough* hormone), known as *hypothyroidism*, your cycles can become shorter, while the period itself is longer with a much heavier flow than normal. Thyroid problems occur in about one in 20 women. If this is the cause of your menstrual irregularity, it is easily remedied. Once your thyroid problem is treated, your periods will simply return to normal.

Finally, irregular cycles may be normal for your age. For example, it often takes young women several years to establish a regular menstrual cycle, and many times, young women will be put on oral contraceptives to regulate their periods. Women beyond 40 can begin menopause at any time, and irregular cycles may be a sign of perimenopause. The term *perimenopause,* which literally means "around menopause," is sometimes used interchangeably with *menopause,* which is clinically the last period of your life — something you cannot know until about a year has passed and you're in postmenopause.

No Menstrual Cycle: Amenorrhea

There is such a thing as having no menstrual cycle, called *amenorrhea.* However, if you don't begin menstruating by the age of 18 there's usually a hormonal imbalance that today is easily remedied with hormonal supplements or oral contraceptives. If you're regularly menstruating and are between 20 and 40, it's unusual to simply stop menstruating. If this does occur, an eating disorder such as anorexia nervosa (food refusal) is the most common cause, as it triggers a protective mechanism in the body.

When the female body is malnourished, it stops ovulating because it can't sustain a pregnancy. One doctor told me about a group of aboriginals in Australia who demonstrate this unique protective mechanism. Women of that particular group only menstruate at certain times of the years, when food is abundant.

Athletes, again, may experience amenorrhea, and both an overactive or underactive thyroid gland, described above, can cause it. (If this is the case, once your thyroid problem is treated you'll begin menstruating again.) In all other cases of a stopped or stunted menstrual cycle, progesterone supplements will remedy it. Natural progesterone therapy is discussed in Chapter 8, "Natural Progesterone Therapy for PMS."

The Need to Bleed

Today, women have to deal with more periods in their lifetime than women did in the past, because of fewer pregnancies and a longer life cycle. Also, in the past century, women have experienced a radical change in their diet, environment, stress levels, and career and family expectations. Understandably, the accumulation of all these factors has affected the hormonal cycle of women, which of course, affects the menstrual cycle.

Again, it's fine to skip a period once in a while, or to experience some occasional fluctuation. But if you've missed more than two periods and you know for certain that you're not pregnant (confirmed by either a pregnancy test or the absence of any sexual activity), then you should investigate having your period induced through a natural progesterone supplement, which will kick-start your cycle again. It's dangerous to go longer than three months without "a bleed"; if the uterus isn't regularly "cleaned out," your risk of uterine cancer can increase.

Heavy Flow: Menorrhagia

An extremely heavy flow may be normal for you. This is known as *primary menorrhagia,* which means that your flow has been heavy since you first began menstruating. If this is the case, there isn't anything to worry about. You should regularly (every six months) have a check-up to make sure your blood count is healthy, however, because consistent heavy flows could cause anemia. In fact, the number one cause of anemia is a heavy menstrual flow.

If a lighter flow slowly *develops* into a continuous heavy flow, this is known as *secondary menorrhagia.* When this happens, as long as you're having annual pelvic exams and biannual blood tests, you shouldn't be concerned. If, however, your flow *suddenly* becomes unexplainably heavy, see your doctor. This kind of *menorrhagia* may signify other problems, such as fibroids or tumors. Flows are considered dangerously heavy if you need to change your pad or tampon every hour.

A Word about Clots

A clot looks like a tiny piece of raw liver or raw oyster, and often comes out with a heavy menstrual flow. Clots are normal and do not mean you're hemorrhaging. Blood naturally clots, and often when you're sleeping during a heavy period, the blood will collect in clots and expel in the morning. The only time you need to worry about clots is if you're passing them after your period is over, during an unusually long period, in midcycle, or while you're pregnant. (Similarly, if you're bleeding at all during these times you should see a doctor.)

When You Experience Abnormally Heavy Bleeding

Abnormally heavy bleeding is when your bleeding is suddenly heavy or significantly heavier than your normal menstrual flow. In fact, it is your own *perception* of what's heavy that's more important than your doctor's perception. And good doctors will try to get you to describe your impression of "heavy" and compare it to your normal pattern. If your doctor tries to determine exactly how much blood you've passed, this is a waste of time for both of you.

Clinically, abnormally heavy menstruation is defined by more than 80 cc's of blood lost per cycle. But studies show that many women who complain of an abnormally heavy flow have lost much less than that. In fact, a more "scientific" measurement is to simply take inventory of the number of pads and tampons you're going through and compare that with your normal pattern.

But Why Is It Suddenly So Heavy?

Your age has a lot to do with your menstrual flow. In fact, teenaged women and women approaching menopause have similar cycles, often characterized by changes in flow. Women between 20 and 40 will have (or should have!) regular patterns that do not fluctuate much from period to period.

If you're under 20 and are noticing heavy bleeding, ask your doctor to check you out for a blood coagulation disorder known as von Willebrand's disease or platelet disorders, such as thrombocytopenia or thrombasthenia.

Most of the time, however, abnormally heavy bleeding is caused by some sort of hormonal disorder, which can be investigated by a reproductive endocrinologist.

If you're over 40, abnormally heavy bleeding is usually caused by what's known as the "anovulatory period." Here, you make estrogen in the first part of your cycle but for some reason (often unknown) you just don't ovulate. Therefore, you do not produce progesterone and you develop an unusually thick uterine lining, which is expelled during your period. This translates into abnormally heavy bleeding.

No matter how old you are, one of the chief culprits of abnormally heavy bleeding in women is high doses of ASA. So if you're fighting off headaches or other ailments before your period, you may want to use an alternative pain reliever.

Sometimes your contraception method can affect your menstrual cycle. For instance, an IUD (intrauterine device) or hormonal contraception can sometimes trigger heavy bleeding. See Chapter 9, "Prescription Drugs Used for PMS," for more details. Changes in exercise patterns (usually less exercise) can also affect your menstrual flow.

What Your Doctor Should Rule Out

If you notice abnormal bleeding either during or between periods, make sure your doctor rules out the following: hyperthyroidism or hypothyroidism (an over- or underactive thyroid gland), ovarian cysts, abnormal tissue within your uterus, as well as endometriosis (discussed further on). Your doctor should also perform a pelvic exam, as well as a transvaginal ultrasound, a procedure in which a dildo-shaped transducer with a condom on it is inserted into your vagina by the ultrasound technician. Transvaginal ultrasound produces much sharper images than abdominal ultrasound.

And, of course, your doctor should be ruling out possible sexually transmitted diseases (STDs).

How Do You Remedy It?

See Chapter 7, "An Herbal and Hands-on Approach," for natural remedies used to treat abnormally heavy bleeding. Natural progesterone therapy is also helpful in regulating flow and cycles, as discussed in Chapter 8. A less invasive traditional medical approach may be taking a nonsteroidal anti-inflammatory drug (NSAID), which will reduce your menstrual flow. A common prescription NSAID is naproxen sodium (such as Anaprox). The usual dose is 275 mg two to four times a day.

If none of these treatments help, you should be evaluated for more serious conditions, such as endometriosis, discussed further on.

Unlike endometriosis, some researchers believe that adenomyosis may set in after pregnancy and delivery; women in their 40s and 50s who have given birth to at least one child are more likely to develop adenomyosis. Other researchers believe that genetics plays a role (like in endometriosis), while some believe that it may have to do with a hormonal imbalance of some sort. The bottom line is that no one knows exactly what causes it, but there are treatments available.

About 40 percent of the time, women have no symptoms, but when they do, the signs are similar to endometriosis: painful and heavy periods and sometimes chronic pelvic pain. Generally, the more involved the uterine glands are, the heavier the flow; the deeper the penetration into the uterine wall, the more discomfort.

Ultrasound followed by laparoscopy is generally the best diagnostic approach available, but often adenomyosis is misdiagnosed as fibroids on the basis of ultrasound tests. As with endometriosis, a laparoscopy is usually the best way to confirm a diagnosis.

Periods on Oral Contraceptives

It's common for younger women, in particular, to be placed on oral contraceptives as a way of controlling their cycles. If you're uncomfortable with taking an oral contraceptive solely for cycle control, and are using another method of birth control, there are natural ways to control your cycle that are discussed further on in this chapter and in Chapter 6, "The Diet and Lifestyle Approach," and Chapter 7, "An Herbal and Hands-on Approach." If you're happy taking an oral contraceptive, as long as you don't smoke and don't have any adverse health problems that oral contraceptives can complicate, you can be on them for a long time if you're regularly monitored by a doctor. There are two kinds of oral contraceptives: combination (these contain synthetic estrogen and progestin, which is a synthetic progesterone) and progestin-only (which contain no estrogen). Oral contraceptives are said to have "noncontraceptive benefits" that include a reduction in ovarian cysts, ovarian cancers, endometrial cancers, and of course, premenstrual discomforts. That's because oral contraceptives stop ovulation. Women who have never been pregnant or breast-fed stand to benefit the most from noncontraceptive benefits, as pregnancy and breast-feeding give your ovaries a natural break from ovulating.

When you are on combination oral contraceptives, your period is chemically induced, called "withdrawal bleeding." On some progestin-only contraception you may also shed the uterine lining once a month. If you're on Depo-Provera or Norplant, your periods are less frequent. Periods on the Pill, as many of us know, are a dream come true: relatively mild cramps, medium-to-light flow, and punctual to the point where you can set your watch by them. For more information on oral contraceptives see Chapter 9, "Prescription Drugs Used for PMS."

Periods after Oral Contraceptives

Many women are surprised to find that when they go off oral contraceptives, their menstrual problems return. If they had irregular cycles before taking oral contraceptives, their cycles will continue to be irregular after they go off the Pill; if they suffered from painful periods before, they will probably have painful periods after; and so on. Oral contraceptives are only a temporary panacea for menstrual cycle problems. Again, you may find more permanent solution to cycle control by reading Chapters 6 and 7. Natural progesterone therapy is also helpful for cycle control, discussed more in Chapter 8, "Natural Progesterone Therapy for PMS."

Some women will continue to have regular cycles when they go off oral contraceptives. This is usually because when they initially went on the Pill, they were younger and had less mature ovulation cycles. Ovulation cycles do mature as we get into our 20s and 30s, which is why the cycles will normalize. But often, as mentioned above, the original cycle — however flawed — returns. Not only is it possible for your original cycle to return (many women actually forget what their true cycle was like), but it can take up to six months for your ovulation cycle to kick in and return to normal. If you're planning to get pregnant, allow at least that much time before you start trying. Doctors will tell you to wait until you get two natural periods before you try to conceive — which is fine — but don't panic if you don't conceive in your third, fourth, or fifth cycle. Many believe that as soon as we go off oral contraceptives we'll get pregnant. This is just not true. Couples having intercourse every other day can wait a year before conception actually takes place.

What to Wear for Your Period

In the early 1990s, women began to be much more aware of products that harmed the environment. For example, washable diapers came back in vogue as a way to reduce our trash. Menstrual products became the focus of much debate when it was learned that plastic tampon applicators are commonly washed up on beaches all over North America because many women flush them and the plastic does not break down in sewage treatment plants. (They are meant to be disposed of in the garbage, which just and the commercial deodorants can irritate your vaginal ecosystem. I list natural ways to deal with the odor at the end of this section. Never use commercially scented tampons or pads; the chemicals used in them can cause irritations and infections.

Don't douche — ever. Douching rids your vagina of friendly bacteria, which are very important for maintaining its ecosystem. Douching is never recommended after menstruation, even though many women practice it. As long you regularly bathe, your vagina and uterus are self-cleaning and will do everything that's necessary on their own. Finally, avoid perfumed or colored toilet paper. Again, the perfumes can irritate your vagina and cause infections.

Natural Ways to Deal with Menstrual and Vaginal Odor

The cheapest natural "odor-eater" during your period is baking soda. Simply bathe in about one cup of baking soda per tubful of water.

Aromatherapy is a wonderful way to smell good below the belt. Purchase essential oil in any health food store. Make sure the label reads: "100% essential oil" or "pure essential oil." Add about six to eight drops of the oil to the bath. A 10- to 20-minute soak in the tub is all you need. Essential oils can be used for all kinds of health problems, including the full range of premenstrual discomforts, allergies, fatigue, depression, and so on (see Chapter 7, "An Herbal and Hands-on Approach"). Depending on the health problem, there are other ways to apply the oils, such as to the soles of the feet, via a diffuser, and so on. But for vaginal odor, sit in a tub! Here are the best oils to have on hand during your period. You can combine them for a real treat, or just use them as single "shots" in the tub.

- **Lavender.** The most useful oil to have on hand as it not only nourishes the female reproductive system and improves vaginal health, but it is also a natural antidepressant and sleep aid.

- **Geranium.** Nourishes the female reproductive system, and has a strong floral scent.

- **Ylang-ylang.** Nourishes the female system and acts as an antidepressant as well as an aphrodisiac! (Try it, you'll like it.)
- **Rose.** Nourishes the female system and also acts as an antidepressant.

If you don't have a bathtub, dilute the oils in a bowl of warm water and use a washcloth or cotton ball to apply the solution as a "wipe" around the vaginal area. This can be done after bowel movements, too, to keep your rectal area nourished and clean.

3

THE EMOTIONAL
PREMENSTRUAL SIGNS

It is the premenstrual emotional changes women experience that have caused women to be diagnosed with the questionable label *premenstrual dysphoric disorder*, discussed in Chapter 1, "PMS Is Not a Disease." Chances are, if you menstruate you experience some of the emotional premenstrual signs described below. The emotional changes are what often wreak havoc on your personal life, and they are also more difficult to link to your periods.

The premenstrual emotional changes women report include some or all of the following:

- Anger (expressed as rage or repressed)
- Anxiety
- Confusion (extremely rare)
- Decreased concentration
- Depression
- Emotional over-responsiveness
- Forgetfulness
- Irritability
- Loss of control
- Melancholy
- Nightmares
- Physical or verbal aggression towards others
- Restlessness
- Sudden mood swings
- Suicidal thoughts (extremely rare)
- Unexplained crying
- Withdrawal

This is a long list! If you think that unexplained behavior and feelings may indeed be caused solely by premenstrual signs, the best thing you can do is *chart* them. Through charting, you'll become more aware of your body and emotions at various stages in the menstrual cycle, which will help you adjust your lifestyle to accommodate for premenstrual mood changes. At the end of this chapter, you'll find a chart I have developed to track mood changes that you can photocopy and freely use as often as you wish. Combine this chart with the one on physical changes in Chapter 4, "The Physical Premenstrual Signs," for a complete story of your premenstrual signs.

Premenstrual mood changes can be classified as emotional or physical (some emotional and physical signs are also called behavioral). Emotional changes (see the chart at the end of this chapter) include irritability, mood swings, anxiety, depression, decreased interest in usual activities, decreased libido, and increased desire to be alone. Physical changes (see the chart in Chapter 4) include increased appetite or food cravings, fatigue, insomnia, hypersomnia (oversleeping), agitation, poor concentration, and poor motor coordination.

If you experience emotional changes premenstrually, there is probably something else going on in your life that is bringing out your emotions at the time of your period. In fact, walking around repressing emotions is far more unhealthy than letting it all out. So the first order of business is looking at *underlying life issues* that probably get aggravated premenstrually. Even if your mood changes completely vanish with the onset of your period, your mood changes are probably not "just PMS." There are social causes for mood changes in women 365 days a year, too! The most recent studies on stress and PMS conclude that PMS is indeed stress-related. That's why understanding the social causes for depression in women is important. We have more stress because of our still-perceived inferior position in our culture. And that can be demoralizing and depressing!

Here's a new thought: Women's bodies may be biologically "set" once a month to express feelings. Tears, in fact, are known to contain high volumes of stress hormones. As unpleasant as we may feel premenstrually, our hormones may be assisting us in ridding ourselves of pent-up feelings that have to get out. Stress hormones block the action of progesterone receptors, too (see Chapter 2 for an explanation of this action). So this may be nature's way of ensuring our reproductive functioning. Think of it as our "premenstrual passion" and it can be a *positive* thing in your life. It is my own theory that passion is normal and healthy; it is the *absence* of passion that is problematic and that is the cause of most depression in women.

Women and Depression

Depression is one of the most notorious emotional signs linked to PMS. Many experts who deal with women and depression note that depression is a "normal" state for women given all of the social problems that still exist for us. As of 1992, women accounted for roughly two-thirds of psychiatric consumers; 84 percent of all psychotherapy patients were reportedly women, while out of all new patients in psychotherapy each year, 60 percent were reportedly women. Statistics from the National Population Health Survey reveal that from 1994 through 1997, 72 percent of reported cases of depression were in women.

In the majority of cases, women suffering from depression have *unipolar depression,* a mood disorder characterized by one low mood. This is distinct from *bipolar depression,* a mood disorder in which there are two moods: one high mood and one low mood.

Most cases of unipolar depression are caused by life circumstances. For this reason, the term "situational depression" is used by mental health care experts to describe most cases of mild, moderate, or even severe unipolar depression in women. A life event can be one trigger of situational depression. Examples of a "life event" include

- Illness
- Job loss or change
- Loss of a loved one (the relationship may have ended or a loved one may have died)
- Moving
- Reproductive life change (childbirth, hysterectomy, or menopause)

Your situational depression may also have been triggered by the *absence* of change in your life, meaning that you are living in a state of continuous struggle, unhappiness, or stress in which no light appears at the end of the tunnel. Examples of "continuous struggle" include

- Abusive relationships
- Body image problems, such as feeling fat or unattractive
- Chronic illness
- Job stress
- Poverty and/or economic worries

A third trigger of situational depression is an absence of resolution regarding past traumas and abuses you suffered as a child or younger woman. Examples of "past traumas" include

- Emotional abuse
- Incest
- Sexual abuse
- Rape
- Violence

In addition, a larger issue of unfair social arrangements still exists for women. In other words, North American culture can chip away at your self-esteem by imposing unfair roles and standards of beauty or ability that can make it hard for you to achieve your personal or professional goals. Many of your "struggles with life" are not your fault; they have to do with the fact that you're a woman living in a 9-to-5 culture that was initially structured for a white male who does not menstruate, get pregnant, breast-feed, or go through menopause. That fact, alone, makes it very hard to get along in this world. But when you factor in other problems, life can get pretty difficult. Our premenstrual hormonal changes are the "icing on the cake" but certainly not the cake!

Violence and Pregnancy.

It's estimated that between 4 and 20 percent (depending on the population studied) of all women will be physically assaulted by a male partner or male ex-partner during their pregnancy. A 1994 report in *the Journal of the American Medical Association* suggests that 37 percent of all obstetrical patients may be abused during pregnancy. In a survey of 6,002 households, it was discovered that a pregnant woman's risk of being abused was 60.6 percent greater than that of nonpregnant woman.

Poverty.

Single women and women of color are far more likely to live in poverty than white men. In 1995, the average income for a Canadian man was $40,419, compared to just $27,624 for a Canadian woman. After a divorce, a man's income increases by roughly 20 percent, yet a woman's income decreases by at least 50 percent. Difficulty with paying bills and making ends meet leads to feelings of anxiousness, sleeplessness, stress, guilt, irritability, and persistent physical symptoms. And poverty is tiring: Many women need to work at two or three jobs in order to survive and cannot afford some of the conveniences that make life easier. This can lead to fatigue, loss of energy, loss of appetite, and so on.

Women in debt are a new spin on poverty — the poverty is often hidden. Many of these women are living in seemingly comfortable surroundings, even though they have "maxed out" their credit cards to pay the rent in between jobs or contracts; are being harassed by creditors; and are one day away from having their car being repossessed. It's also important to note that many women in poverty or debt are also the "hidden homeless," even though they are not visible on the streets. Untold numbers of women camp out on the couches of friends and relatives, looking for employment or a place to live.

Workplace Stress and Harassment.

Even though it's the 21st century, women still must cope with sexual harassment, ageism, and sexism in the workplace, which often leads to loss of employment. Those women forced to work two jobs to make ends meet can be exposed to twice the abuse on the job in the form of harassment or stress. As well, they experience plain old stress caused by the long hours and commuting that *all* people in the workplace endure. See Chapter 4, "The Physical Premenstrual Signs," for more details on stress.

Beauty Standards.

Impossible standards of beauty are another factor that makes life difficult for women. Aside from body image anxiety, physical symptoms caused by any resulting eating disorders can cause restlessness, irritability, difficulty concentrating or making decisions, loss of interest in formerly pleasurable activities, and feelings of self-doubt and self-hatred.

Illness.
A related factor in many cases of depression is chronic illness. Women living with arthritis, osteoporosis, colitis, HIV/AIDS, cancer, and other chronic diseases can experience many of the symptoms associated with depression, such as loss of appetite, sleeplessness, and loss of interest in formerly pleasurable activities. To aggravate matters, medications, ranging from chemotherapy to AZT, used in a variety of situations, can cause depression as well.

Infertility.
Roughly 20 percent of Canadian couples are infertile. A study done by Harvard professor Dr. Alice Domar found that women who were undergoing fertility treatment experienced levels of depression that equaled those of women facing cancer or AIDS. First, the circumstance of infertility, by itself, can trigger all the feelings and symptoms associated with biological depression. Meanwhile, the hormonal changes created by fertility drugs can also trigger biological depression and badly aggravate PMS. Estrogen functions as a weak antidepressant, and when fertility drugs are introduced, your mood can head south. Then, the cost of treatment can place such a strain on your finances, it's, well ... depressing. There is also grief involved with being diagnosed as infertile, as women tend to mourn for their unborn children and must accept a change in identity from "mother-to-be" to "childless woman."

Pregnancy Loss.
Pregnancy loss is a common trigger for depression in women of childbearing age. One in six pregnancies ends in miscarriage, but as women age, the miscarriage rate increases. Women who have struggled with infertility also miscarry at higher rates.

Divorce.
Whether you were living common-law or were married, the dissolution of a long-term relationship with an intimate partner leads to feelings of grief, sadness, loneliness, isolation, and often financial hardship: all fodder for a depressive episode.

Feeling Unconnected

The large body of work that looks at causes of sadness and depression shows us that people suffer most when they are feeling unconnected with the world around them.

When women talk informally to try and put their feelings into perspective, these are some of the things they talk about:

- **Sexism.** In case you haven't noticed, we live in a sexist society where men still enjoy more privileges than women. Ask other women how they feel about that. Your conversation won't change the world, but your feelings about the world might be validated. And that feels good.

- **Powerlessness.** You know what? You feel powerless because you're "set up" to feel powerless — by those in power! Most women have very little power in their workplace, home, community, and so forth. So it's no wonder you feel inadequate. Talking about this may help you find a perspective that actually empowers you. By the way, this is not to say that there are no powerful women in the world; it's just that they are few and far between. And there are plenty of women in power who feel powerless, too.

- **Ambivalence over assertiveness.** I know it's the 21st century, but women in many cultures are taught to be docile and passive in a world that is aggressive and harsh. Again, talking about it won't necessarily change you into a "go-getter," but it will probably help you realize that you're not the only one out there who has been taught to feel that aggressiveness and assertiveness are unfeminine. Therefore, your reluctance to assert yourself is perfectly understandable, given the message you're sent from birth: you do not have a voice and when you speak, negative consequences follow.

- **Absurd standards of beauty.** Spend an afternoon with a fashion photographer and make-up artist, and they can tell you a few things. What you see in the magazines is fiction and fantasy with the aid of heavy makeup, carefully constructed lighting, and computer-aided touch-ups. In fact, it's common for fashion models to self-induce vomiting prior to a photo shoot (the make-up artists can smell the vomit on the model while she's in make-up). Is that beautiful? Talk about *that* with other women! One make-up artist put it best when he told me: "I can't even watch television or read a magazine anymore because I know how ugly this business is, and how desperate the women are who participate in this sham. We [make-up artists and photographers] spend hours distorting these women and dare call it 'beauty.'"

When it is the Caucasian face that is objectified and held up as the global standard of beauty, what are you supposed to do if you're not Caucasian? Does this standard of beauty make sense to you? And when 17-year-old girls are objectified and held up as the standard for what a 35-year-old woman is supposed to look like, isn't that *insane*? Models (who must be at least 5'9" to get work) are taller than the average *Caucasian* woman. So if you're of average height for a Caucasian, you're not considered beautiful ▶

enough for the Western standard. But of course, most women on the planet are not Caucasian. The average height for Asian women, for example, is shorter than the average Caucasian height. Again, our beauty standards are not sane.

When we feel "plugged in" to our community and network of friends and colleagues, we feel increased zest, well-being, and motivation. Connection brings us increased self-worth, as well as a desire to make more connections. The flip side of wanting to connect with someone is that we can open up too much and become vulnerable. Vulnerability can, of course, lead us to be taken advantage of. Most people have a few bitter experiences of their vulnerability and openness allowing less than savory characters into their lives. A lot of us may stray into relationships with people who take terrible advantage of our feelings and openness. The problem with vulnerability is that it cannot be halfway. There is simply no way around this risk. This is why many of us learn to shut down; this is when passion becomes repressed, predisposing us to depression or numbness.

Cutting ourselves off from people can also cause loneliness. Solitude is rejuvenating; loneliness is stressful. Loneliness comes from a lack of truly intimate relationships with friends or family members; intimacy, in this case, refers to sharing deep feelings, fears, and so on with someone. This is how we unburden ourselves and relieve stress. Feeling as though you belong somewhere, or feeling part of a community, can also alleviate loneliness. Here are steps you can take to create more supportive relationships in your life:

- Find some sort of social group to belong to by looking into gourmet cooking clubs, art classes, and so on. Find an activity that you're really drawn to, and chances are, you'll meet like-minded souls with whom you can form quality friendships.

- Have a couple of nice dinner parties each year. It's a way to create more intimate friendships with people who may only be acquaintances or casual friends.

- Get involved in your community. Whether it's a "not in my backyard" lobby or a community street sale, get out and meet your neighbors. Participating in community-based programs, ranging from crafts groups to yoga, is the way to gain support. In fact, community outreach workers use the arts, crafts, fitness, and computer classes, and so on, as a tool to attract people in the community who

could benefit from support. What often takes place in community-based programs is a great deal of talking and sharing during, prior to, or after the activity.
These are places where you make friends; find someone you can talk to; and most
importantly, find that you're not alone

- Volunteer. Volunteering for causes dear to your heart is a great way to meet people and feel needed. Meals on wheels, eldercare facilities, street youth programs,
  and so forth all attract wonderful souls with whom you may find friendship and
  comfort.

- Get a dog. Dogs need to be walked, which means you'll meet other people walking their dogs. And dog owners tend to gravitate toward other dog owners. It's a
  great jumping-off point for meeting people. Aside from that, many studies point
  to the health effects of pet ownership, including lowered blood pressure and lowered incidences of heart disease. (Positive health effects can be seen with any pet,
  including cats!)

Learning to Express Anger

Women in our culture are not allowed to openly express their anger, unless it's in the
interest of someone or something else: a child, a partner, or a cause. Many women
turn it inward, and their repressed anger manifests as depression. When this doesn't
happen, the anger becomes misdirected and confused, spawning all kinds of negative
behaviors and relationships.

Common manifestations of women's anger include

- **Depression.** Depression in women is commonly understood as "anger turned
  inward." Anger is mobilizing; depression is immobilizing.

- **Eating disorders.** See Chapter 6, "The Diet and Lifestyle Approach," for more
  details.

- **Self-harm.** This is a broad category that includes harmful addictions, harmful
  relationships, suicide attempts, self-mutilation, and self-destructive or self-
  sabotaging behaviors.

- **Harming others.** This broad category includes petty crimes, such as theft; "vexa-
  tious lies" (lies that deliberately hurt versus "white lies"); harassment (stalking,
  repeated phone calls or e-mails); violence against children (women's powerlessness can be turned against those with even less power — their children); and
  heinous crimes (murder, or extreme violence against others).

Why We Can't Get Angry

Because women grow up in this society in a subordinate role, we can develop an inner belief system that makes it difficult to express anger. Many women believe the following:

- I am weak. If I express my anger, I'll be overpowered.
- I am dependent. If I express my anger, I may disrupt my lifestyle.
- I have no right to feel anger. If I express my anger, I won't be liked or loved as much. (This belief is an extension of feelings of low self-worth and self-esteem.)
- I want people to think I'm nice. I don't want to be labeled a "bitch" or a "nag" or "bitter." (This belief stems from negative stereotypes associated with angry women.)

Women also suffer when they feel they are disconnected to the world around them. Therefore, anger may threaten to sever their relationships, and so they may go to great lengths to mask their anger. Many women rank having a relationship as more valuable than having a "self." As a result, terms such as "de-selfing" and "silencing of the self" are used in academic articles and books focusing on women and anger. De-selfing or silencing of the self means that your whole value system (what you think, want, etc.) is "up for sale" in order to keep the peace in your relationships. The flip side is that when we do this long enough, we become very angry. De-selfing, or silencing of self, is considered to be at the root of most women's inability to express anger.

Ruling out Seasonal Affective Disorder (SAD)

I'm sure by now you've read a lot about seasonal affective disorder (SAD). This is a fairly recent label that came into use in 1987, even though mood disorders have long been known to be triggered by changes in seasons. SAD typically strikes women in their 20s and 30s, and is seen more in regions at higher latitudes. The person with SAD will notice atypical symptoms of depression during the winter, when she sleeps too much and eats too much (thereby gaining weight). Then she begins to "wake up" in the spring and can even be slightly manic (known as hypomanic). (Occasionally, the reverse occurs, and the symptoms of major depression present themselves during the summer months, instead. This may be related to extreme discomfort in humid, hot weather, inability to sleep as a result, increased pollutants in the air, and all the other miseries of humid, hot urban summers.) In short, SAD has many of the features of hibernation — oversleeping and "storing up" on fat or carbohydrates for the cold winter. It's "bear and squirrel" behavior in humans, which can be debilitating.

Living or working in areas that are light-deprived can also lead to SAD. For example, people who spend weeks or months at a time on submarines exhibit symptoms of SAD. And here's a true urban tale: A friend of mine developed a bad case of SAD when she moved into a basement apartment without windows. Since she was looking for a cheap "crash pad" for a couple of months while she was in a transition period, she was looking for something serviceable and didn't consider the "no window" factor a problem. It was. Within a couple of weeks, she began craving sweets and junk food like mad, and became quite blue, irritable, and apathetic: she was depressed. Several friends commented that she should move to a place with *windows*. And she did. Her symptoms vanished within about a week, and she was amazed at how dramatically her basement flat had affected her mood.

Treating SAD

Light at the end of the tunnel is in sight for women with SAD — literally. Light can be like a drug. If you've been diagnosed with SAD, you may be prescribed light rather than pills (medications may also be effective). Often, the "cure" for SAD is to re-create the kind of light you'd naturally be exposed to on a nice summer's day. Sitting under your chandelier won't do. You need to be sitting in front of bright, full-spectrum fluorescent or incandescent lights for about 30–120 minutes in order for this to work. It's not necessary to have sunlight or sun-like light. To protect your eyes, the lights are covered with a sheer material. You can get the light you need with a "light box." Just do whatever you like in front of these lights. You'll need to sit close — which is only about a foot and a half away.

In order for light treatment to work, you need to keep your eyes open, so napping isn't a good thing. If you prefer to sleep, there is an experimental device known as a dawn simulator, which can work while you sleep. Most people start to feel better in a few days of 30-minute-per-day light treatments.

Even this treatment has some side effects: mild headaches or eyestrain are not unusual, and sometimes mild mania (from the production of serotonin) may even occur. If you're taking a drug that makes you sensitive to bright light, you are not a good candidate for this therapy. See your doctor for information on purchasing a light box.

Bright light therapy has also been shown to help depression that isn't necessarily SAD, but is necessarily related to what's known as circadian rhythm sleep disorders (that is, sleep disorders involving your "biological clock"). In this case, light therapy during the day has been shown to help with sleep problems.

The message of seeking comfort in validation and treatment for your depression is not to confirm your suspicions that life is "horrible and hopeless," but to show you that you're not the only one who feels life is a struggle. This should give you the courage to move forward and make some changes (or at least, make some friends who have common concerns) instead of shrinking in a corner feeling you're the "only one."

Managing Mood Changes Anytime of the Month

Regardless of when in your cycle you experience mood changes, finding someone to talk to can make a world of difference. Combining talk therapy with natural healing strategies discussed in Chapters 6 and 7 is the best formula for stabilizing your mood. Antidepressants should be looked at as a last resort (see Chapters 1 and 9).

When you're looking for a therapist, you should focus on finding someone you can relate to and who is a "good fit." The pitfall you want to avoid is winding up with a therapist who is not helpful. Unhelpful therapy does not mean that your therapist is a poor or unethical therapist; it means that the style of therapy is not well suited to you, and/or your therapist is not someone with whom you feel entirely comfortable. There can be many reasons for this, and they are often difficult to nail down. In other words, the therapy one woman finds helpful another woman may not. Therapists and styles of therapies are highly individual and so is their impact.

The following are some ways to find a therapist.

Employee Assistance Programs.

These are programs many workplaces now offer. The employer prepays a group of therapists for a certain number of hours of therapy. You call a toll-free number completely confidentially, whereupon you have the option of seeing various licensed therapists on a short-term basis. Some therapists may specialize more in addiction or stress management, while others may specialize in depression. This is relatively "risk-free" in that if you don't like the person you see, you simply don't go back. And it has not cost you anything.

Community Family Services or Women's Health Clinics.

Some communities operate family and child services, or women's clinics, where you can call to book an appointment with a staff social worker who can help you. In some cases, you may be able to drop in unannounced, but calling ahead of time is always best. These services are usually not free, but you will be charged according to your ability to pay.

Crisis Lines.

If you're feeling overwhelmed and need to speak to somebody right away, calling a crisis telephone line, listed in the front of your white pages, is an option. A crisis counselor can also refer you to other people or places for more long-term counseling.

Community Services Listings.

Most urban areas have a publication that lists community services or, at least, a list of community services phone numbers. (Ontario, for example, has a "Blue Book" with such listings.) You can find these in public libraries.

Friends.

You may or may not feel comfortable going to a therapist recommended by a friend. Confidentiality would be the main concern, but if you trust your friend and see that she or he has been helped by a particular therapist, you may feel good about going to this professional. As noted, successful therapy is so personal that most experts in mental health will tell you *not* to use "hairdresser rules" for therapists, but it often depends on the circumstances. You should be careful about "gurus" or people who seem to have tremendous influence on the friend who has been helped. There are a variety of "cult-like" therapists who have no formal training and who practice dangerous mind games and brainwashing on the vulnerable.

Looking for Credentials

When you're shopping for a therapist, one of the most confusing words is "doctor" because it can mean either the person is a medical doctor or has a Ph.D., which stands for "doctor of philosophy." People obtain Ph.D.'s in a number of academic disciplines ranging from *A* (as in anthropology) to *Z* (as in zoology). Furthermore, just because someone is a trained medical doctor doesn't mean he or she is a psychiatrist, or a trained therapist, either.

An interesting example of credential confusion is the education of Dr. Laura Schlessinger, who hosts a popular internationally syndicated radio show. Most people assume that Dr. Laura is either a psychologist or a psychiatrist. But if you look at her credentials, you'll see that she obtained her Ph.D. in physiology and is said to hold "postdoctoral certification and licensing in marriage and family therapy." This means that Dr. Laura did not earn her Ph.D. in the area of mental health. It does not mean she isn't qualified, however, for after completing her Ph.D., she indeed took the same certification courses taken by many other therapists, who do not necessarily hold

Ph.D.'s. But because we can slide "doctor" in front of her name, the power of the title suggests she holds more credentials in the field of therapy than she actually does.

Even the "right" letters don't mean that a therapist is properly trained in therapy. For example, a social worker who has a Master of Social Work (MSW) could obtain such a degree by taking some general courses in social work theory, but may not have any training specifically related to counseling or therapy. Or a social worker may have spent most of his or her professional life in policy jobs, with no exposure to counseling or therapy. Letters may also be meaningless if that therapist obtained them through a disreputable university, college, or society.

But looking at letters is certainly a start, helping you to sort out what sort of training your therapist has likely received. The following professionals should have the corresponding credentials.

Psychiatrist.

A psychiatrist is a medical doctor who specializes in the medical treatment of mental illness and is able to prescribe drugs. Many psychiatrists also do psychotherapy, but this isn't always the case. The appropriate credentials should read: Jane Doe, M.D. (medical doctor), F.R.C.P. (Fellow, Royal College of Physicians). That means this doctor has gone through four years of medical school and has completed a residency program in psychiatry, which, depending on the province, lasted approximately four years, and is registered in the Royal College of Physicians and Surgeons.

Psychologist and Psychological Associate.

A psychologist or psychological associate is someone who is licensed to practice therapy with either a master's degree or doctoral degree. Clinical psychologists have a Master of Science (MSc.) or Master of Arts (MA), and will usually work in a hospital or clinic setting, but often can be found in private practice. Clinical psychologists can also hold a Ph.D. (Doctor of Philosophy) in psychology, an Ed.D. (Doctor of Education) or, if they're American, a Psy.D. (Doctor of Psychology), a common degree in the United States. Psychologists often perform testing, make assessments, and plan treatments. They can also do psychotherapy, may have hospital admitting privileges, and should be registered in the College of Psychologists. In most provinces, people calling themselves "psychologists" would have to be registered or licensed by a provincial body, which isn't necessarily meaningful unless the psychologist worked in a certain kind of setting. The problem with licenses is that you could have someone who is well-trained as a psychotherapist, with a Ph.D. in psychology, who isn't registered with the province, while someone with no training who is an experimental psychologist, for example (having, say, spent most her professional life with white mice), could call herself registered. In some states in the United States, psychologists can also prescribe drugs (in case you seek out help while spending time in the United States).

Social Worker.

This professional holds a BSW (Bachelor of Social Work) and/or a MSW (Master of Social Work), having completed a bachelor's degree in another discipline (which is not at all uncommon). Some social workers have a Ph.D. as well. The designation CSW stands for Certified Social Worker, a designation given by the College of Social Work to say that this person is certified and meets the standards to be a member of the College. In order to obtain a CSW, exams and supervision are required. Social workers can provide counseling and psychotherapy, but it's important to ask your social worker what specific training she or he has had in the area of mental health.

Psychiatric Nurse.

A psychiatric nurse is most likely a registered nurse (RN) with a Bachelor of Science degree (BSc.) in nursing (which isn't absolutely required) who probably has, but doesn't necessarily require, a master's degree in nursing, too. The master's degree could be either an MA (Master of Arts) or an MSc. (Master of Science). This nurse has done most of his or her training in a psychiatric setting, and *may* be trained to do psychotherapy.

Counselor.

This professional has *usually* completed certification courses in counseling and therefore has obtained a license to practice psychotherapy; she or he may have, but does not require, a university degree. Frequently, though, counselors will have a master's degree in a related field, such as social work. Or they may have a master's degree in a field having nothing to do with mental health. The bad news is that there are no official credentials required by a counselor, in that there is no legal regulation of the term. Nevertheless, while a television repair person can, *in theory*, set up a counseling practice, it's unlikely you'll encounter this. There are various provincial societies and associations to which counselors may belong, but association, membership, and/or affiliation has little to do with this professional's skill as a therapist. For example, a counselor's business card in Toronto may state that she is a member of the Ontario Society of Psychotherapy. That doesn't mean that she is a good psychotherapist, but it does mean that there are some standards of practice that she is upholding in order to be a member. It's always a good idea to ask your counselor what training she has had in the field of mental health.

Marriage and Family Counselor.

A marriage or family counselor is somewhat different from the broader term "counselor." This professional has completed rigorous training through certification courses in family therapy and relationship dynamics, and has obtained a license to practice psychotherapy. This professional may or may not have a master's degree or Ph.D. in a related field. This professional should have designations such as OAFMT (Ontario Association of Family and Marital Therapy) or AAFMT (American Association of Family and Marital Therapy).

A Word about Fees

It's important to discuss fees with your therapist up front, so you know what services the province or your health plan covers, and which fees are not covered. In general, the province covers mental health services in hospitals and services provided by psychiatrists. But social workers or counselors in private practice are all fee-for-service. Call your provincial College of Social Work to determine what a social worker or counselor in private practice should be charging. If you want to see someone in private practice but can't afford to pay, community-provided counseling services are based on your ability to pay. Experts consulted for this book agreed that it is considered bad practice for a counselor to agree to see someone who cannot (or will not) pay for his or her services. This person is offering a service, not a charity, and the professional relationship should be respected.

Going for a Test Drive

Okay. You found someone you think is qualified to be your therapist. That doesn't mean you found the right therapist for *you*. Ask yourself the following questions when you first sit down with this therapist. If you find you answer "no" to many of the questions below, you should ask yourself whether you're really with the right therapist. There is no magic number of "no's" here; but these questions will help you gauge how you truly feel about this therapist.

1. Is this someone you feel comfortable with?

2. Is this someone you can trust?

3. Is this someone you feel calm with?

4. Is this someone you feel safe with?

5. Does this person respect you (or treat you with respect)?

6. Does this person seem flexible?

7. Does this person seem reliable?

8. Does this person seem supportive?

9. Does this person have a supervisor or mentor with whom they consult on difficult or challenging cases?

Red Flags

You should be cautious about engaging a therapist in the following scenarios:

- She or he does not do a formal assessment, known as a work-up, that includes ruling out organic causes for your moods, such as thyroid disease, for example. If your therapist is not a physician, she or he may not be trained to do a complete physical exam as a physician would do, but may still be an excellent therapist. However, a therapist *should* ask you where you've been prior to this appointment, and at least inquire about whether you've had a physical exam.

- If you're seeing a medical doctor or psychiatrist and she or he prescribes antidepressants or other medications during your first visit. (See Chapter 5, "Finding a PMS Doctor.") As a general rule, some sort of work-up and discussion is necessary before you're handed a prescription and sent home.

- You are "diagnosed" or "labeled" with a disorder of some sort within a few minutes of your first visit. This is a situation that would only occur if your therapist is a medical doctor. You may be clearly suffering from an identifiable mood disorder, but some discussion and work-up should be happening before you're diagnosed.

- She or he is adamantly opposed to prescribing any sort of medication, no matter what. (This isn't good, either; some people require medication *and* talk therapy).

- She or he believes in only one kind of approach or theory and seems inflexible to any other approach, theory, or school of thought, such as a woman-centered approach. This is okay if the therapist is clear and open about the fact that she or he believes in only one approach, explains to you why she or he believes it's helpful, and points out the limitations of her or his work. In this case, you've been informed about the pros and cons and are free to decide whether the one-school-of-thought approach is for you.

- She or he does not ask you about your relationships, school and work histories, or other aspects of your personal history.

- She or he uses a lot of complicated jargon or technical language that intimidates you. How can you possibly expect to talk to someone when you can't understand what she or he is saying?

- She or he suggests you have sex with her or him to work through your sexual problems. This is malpractice and should be reported. And yes, women can abuse women, although it is rare.

Does the Age or Lifestyle of Your Therapist Matter?

The only time the age or lifestyle of your therapist matters is if it matters to *you*, because it will affect your degree of comfort with that therapist. Although younger therapists certainly have less life experience than older therapists, everyone knows there are just as many wise 31-year-olds as there are 56-year-olds with little wisdom. Younger therapists may be more flexible, caring, less "burnt out," and more up-to-date in terms of codes of practice and ethics. Older therapists may have more experience, but may also be more rigid in their approach. Older therapists may be more sensitive to fears of death or aging than a younger therapist. Meanwhile, a childless therapist may be less apt to understand the stresses of a woman with children. Gender preference may also be a factor. If you're a lesbian, you may be more comfortable with a therapist who is gay or lesbian.

However, finding someone who is similar to you in some ways because you want the feeling of automatic acceptance isn't a guarantee that this is the right therapist. Other dynamics are also important; you may be uncomfortable with a father figure, for example, or a mother figure; you may be equally uncomfortable with someone the same age as your son or daughter. Although most people strive to find a "peer" in a therapist, a therapist and client are not "equal" in this context. In other words, looking for a therapist who is like yourself may not be the best criterion when you're looking for a therapist because there is enormous value in finding a person with the right therapeutic distance.

Styles of Therapy

There are many styles of therapy and therapists out there. The following are the styles most useful if you suffer from PMS.

Feminist Therapy

Feminist therapy means "woman-centered therapy." Feminist therapy is not one specific style of therapy, but an overall philosophy of therapy that takes women's social roles and social situations into account when looking at the symptoms that compose women's depression. This is especially key when you're coping with emotional mood changes associated with your period. Careful: I am not saying this is the *only* approach to therapy. And plenty of female therapists do *not* embrace feminist therapy. The following goals represent a feminist approach to therapy:

- Developing a sense of self, independent of male authority or idealized visions of what a woman is supposed to be; the task is not to for a woman to develop a "male persona" but to celebrate her own feminine persona and to see her traits as inner strength rather than an inability to compete in a male world.

- Seeing that the "personal is political," as the adage goes. Feminist therapists listen for the connections between the personal story and the outer world in women's lives. The therapist uses feminist values to help shift a woman from a "victim" into a person who sees how the world *around* her is creating her feelings of victimization — which is therefore validating.

- Seeing that depression is really the internalization of oppression. (This does not mean, however, that you should just walk around depressed and not seek out help.)

- Seeing that feelings of low self-esteem, worthlessness, inadequacy, powerlessness, poor body image, anxiety, depression, and/or sexual dysfunction are symptoms of female subservience in a man's world. In other words, they are normal, adaptive responses to the world around you, rather than symptoms of a disease or sickness. (Again, this does not mean that you should just "shrug off" your feelings of depression, low self-esteem, and so on, and not get help. In other words, cold symptoms may be normal reactions to a common cold virus, but you still need to care for yourself by resting and drinking plenty of fluids to get better.)

- Seeing that self-sacrificing behaviors are normal feminine, nurturing behaviors rather than symptoms of a disease. Labels such as "co-dependent" are not helpful and should be dismissed as "psychobabble."

- Seeing that physical ailments are valid and should be trusted as another way of "knowing." In other words, women's bodies may be trying to "tell" them something about the environment or the toxic lifestyle to which they have become numb. For example, many women who have chronic fatigue or environmental sensitivities should see their symptoms as visionary or intuitive, rather than invalid and phantom. There is a link between feminine intuition, ecology, and environment, which feminists have called "eco-feminism." Women such as Rachel Carson, author of *Silent Spring*, who warned of the dangers of pesticides as early as 1964 and was declared a heretic by the pharmaceutical industry, are examples of how women's physical ailments and body intuition were dismissed to the world's peril.

- Seeing that human emotional pain is not a medical problem but a normal response to one's environment. In other words, pain in response to a bad situation, is normal, not sick.

- Understanding that grief is grief. Grieving over the death of a loved one is not different from grieving over one's poverty or life circumstances. Yet, in the medical world, some things are more worthy of grief than others, meaning that you are labeled normal for some kinds of grieving but "sick" for other kinds.

- Connecting to other women as a group. What you suffer, other women suffer. You are not alone, but part of a community. The solution cannot be found on an individual level, but must be arrived at collectively. In other words, one black person in 1950 could not overturn centuries of racism and segregation. It took a movement.

A therapist doesn't have to be a female to offer a woman-centered approach. If you are interested in seeking help with a feminist therapist, the best places to contact for names are women's centers or even women's studies programs at local universities. Alternatively, use the guidelines for finding help earlier in this chapter and simply tell your therapist that you are interested in a *feminist approach*.

Cognitive-Behavioral Therapy

Cognitive-behavioral therapy is oriented toward upbeat thinking and correcting what is referred to as "disordered thinking." Instead of dwelling on negative thoughts, this form of therapy is based on the premise that "how you think can affect how you feel." For example, if a friend cancels a lunch date with you, or somebody doesn't return your phone call or e-mail, you may be apt to take it personally and assume that you are not liked by that person. That thought then leads you to feel badly about yourself, reinforcing feelings of low self-esteem or even self-loathing. A cognitive-behavioral therapist will ask you to consider other reasons for the cancellation or unreturned call. Perhaps there are other problems overwhelming that person that have absolutely nothing to do with you. Perhaps a last-minute deadline came up, or problems and stresses in your lunch date's personal life necessitated the cancellation. In other words, not everything you perceive to be negative is really negative; and not everything you take personally is personal.

Ultimately, the premise of cognitive-behavioral therapy is this: If you think negative thoughts about yourself and believe you're a failure, or that your life is doomed, you are more apt to be sad. On the other hand, if you think positive thoughts and believe in yourself, you are more apt to be happy. Although this approach might sound "easy" and "quick-fix," changing your perspective on life can be powerful. But again, in the midst of a depression, this approach may have limited success. Essentially, what's past is past, and you can decide *today* to be a more positive person, which in turn, can attract more positive experiences into your life.

Interpersonal Therapy

Interpersonal therapy is a very specific approach based on the idea that malfunctioning relationships are the source of your depression, mood swings, or lifestyle stresses. In other words, where there are such problems, there are "screwed-up" relationships in your life that are interfering with your quality of life. You and your therapist will explore current relationships and recent events that may have affected those relationships, such as loss, conflict, or change. You may also explore the roles various people are playing in your life and what your expectations are of them, and vice versa. Your therapist works in a supporting role to help you to develop better strategies to cope or negotiate with key people in your life, which can help to resolve conflicts. Much of this approach has to do with setting reasonable expectations from relationships, and looking at how you might have misinterpreted actions of others.

Psychodynamic Therapy

Psychodynamic therapy deals with the "ghosts" or relationships and events from your past, the dynamics of your upbringing, as well as present events and relationships. Here, your thoughts, emotions, and behavior over a lifetime are examined, and patterns of behavior and aspects of your personality are discussed as possible sources of both internal and external conflict. Couples or groups are often involved in psychodynamic therapy. The adage "the past is history, the future a mystery, and the present a gift" works well in this context.

Biologically Informed Psychotherapy

If you believe you need antidepressants, biologically informed psychotherapy is another approach, known as "biopsychiatry." Here, your therapist believes depression is a medical problem, triggered by some life pressure or stressor. Medication combined with talk therapy is the preferred approach, and if you are believed to suffer from seasonal depression, light therapy may be used instead of medication.

This doesn't mean your therapist is against "talk therapy," however. She or he may combine one of the styles of therapy discussed above in addition to medication. But instead of seeing your depression as stemming solely from a social situation, a therapist who practices biopsychiatry will see your "depressive thinking," for example, as a side-effect of depression, which is viewed as a medical condition. If you are thinking about suicide, rather than look at your personal situation or life events triggering this thought or desire, a therapist from this "school" would say: "That's your depression talking (that is, your disordered brain chemistry), not *you*." Thus, your depression is removed from your circumstances, and treated like a medical condition, such as pneumonia. The belief is that once your brain chemistry is "restored" you will begin to think rationally and reasonably again, may even be able to shift your perspective on life, which could be done through talk therapy.

This is not unlike an approach used to treat anorexia nervosa, for example. A woman suffering from anorexia may benefit enormously from talk therapy. But if she weighs under 60 pounds and is physically starving, there is no way for her to "hear" what is being said, let alone participate in talk therapy. She will therefore need to be fed and be physically "restored" before she can hear anything. If you are incapacitated by your depression, for example, and cannot get out of bed, talk therapy is not useful; the main goal of your therapist in this case would be to help you *get out of bed*, and thus "restore" your functioning. This may be done through medications, such as antidepressants (see Chapter 9, "Prescription Drugs Used for PMS").

Biopsychiatry does not mean that the therapist believes medication will "fix" everything; simply that it can facilitate productive talk therapy.

Psychoanalysis

It's important not to confuse psychoanalysis with psychoanalytic therapy, which is more along the lines of psychodynamic therapy. Psychoanalysis is an intensive therapy that usually involves daily sessions, and is not recommended for people in the midst of a depression, where you are not able to function well. This therapy is best when the crisis has passed, and is therapy designed for people ready for self-discovery. It is a journey into your childhood based on the premise that problems you have today stem from deep wounds from your childhood. For example, you may be re-enacting unmet needs you had as a child in your adult life. Or you may discover that behavior such as "pleasing your parents" is being acted out in your workplace or in your personal relationships. In previous books, I've discussed how women in the past were frequently harmed through psychoanalysis because it tended to reinforce father figure/little-girl relationships. But properly done, it is not something women have to fear, and many excellent psychoanalysts are women.

Charting Emotional Premenstrual Signs

Use the chart below to help you determine when in your cycle your mood changes begin, end, "peak and valley." Remember that Day 1 of your cycle is the first day of bleeding, or day 1 of your period.

My Emotional Cycle Chart

Cycle Day: **Calendar Date:**

Check the boxes to the left that represent the feelings, perceptions, or experiences you have today. Circle the number on the right to rate the degree to which you feel/perceive/experience these things. 10 means "very severe" and 1 means "very mild."

	Very mild							Very severe		
[ ] Aggression	1	2	3	4	5	6	7	8	9	10
[ ] Anger (expressed as rage or repressed)	1	2	3	4	5	6	7	8	9	10
[ ] Anxiety	1	2	3	4	5	6	7	8	9	10
[ ] Confusion	1	2	3	4	5	6	7	8	9	10
[ ] Decreased concentration	1	2	3	4	5	6	7	8	9	10
[ ] Depression	1	2	3	4	5	6	7	8	9	10
[ ] Forgetfulness	1	2	3	4	5	6	7	8	9	10
[ ] Irritability	1	2	3	4	5	6	7	8	9	10
[ ] Loss of control	1	2	3	4	5	6	7	8	9	10
[ ] Melancholy	1	2	3	4	5	6	7	8	9	10
[ ] Overreacting	1	2	3	4	5	6	7	8	9	10
[ ] Restlessness	1	2	3	4	5	6	7	8	9	10
[ ] Suicidal thoughts	1	2	3	4	5	6	7	8	9	10
[ ] Sudden mood swings	1	2	3	4	5	6	7	8	9	10
[ ] Unexplained crying	1	2	3	4	5	6	7	8	9	10
[ ] Withdrawal	1	2	3	4	5	6	7	8	9	10

Describe your dreams.

If you can remember your dreams, describe them here. Dreams change according to the cycle and can be valuable clues to what you are working on in your "inner life." Pick up a dream dictionary to help you with symbols.

_____

_____

_____

What did you eat today?

Moods can be linked to blood sugar swings. List your meals and snacks and times you ate them.

_____

_____

_____

Special circumstances

Did anything out of the ordinary occur today? If so, explain:

_____

_____

_____

Moon cycle

Take note of the moon's position so you can chart your emotional changes in accordance with moon changes. Remember, the Greek word for "moon" is _mene_, while _menstruation_ actually means "moon change." Chart any eclipses and so on.

_____

_____

_____

Emotional Cycle Chart, Copyright © M. Sara Rosenthal, 2001.

THE PHYSICAL PREMENSTRUAL SIGNS

4

In the previous chapter, we looked at underlying social causes for depression, anxiety, anger, and the host of premenstrual emotions and mood changes that women experience. Many of you discovered from reading Chapter 3 that there are *other* things going on in your life that "crash" into your premenstrual changes. If you can try to solve some of the underlying problems affecting your life, many of you will see dramatic changes to your moods around your period. The same thing applies to physical changes.

This list isn't exhaustive, but women report the following physical premenstrual signs:

- Abdominal bloating (which may also cause weight gain)
- Acne or other skin eruptions
- Asthma
- Backache
- Breast swelling and tenderness
- Changes in sex drive (either more or less)
- Chills, shakiness, and dizziness
- Clumsiness and poor coordination
- Constipation or diarrhea
- Eye problems
- Fatigue
- Headaches
- Heart pounding
- Hoarseness
- Increased appetite and weight gain
- Insomnia
- Joint and muscle pain
- Menopausal-like hot flashes
- Nausea
- Seizures
- Sensitivity to noise
- Sugar and salt cravings

Yet another long list! When looking at the physical changes women experience premenstrually, it's important to rule out underlying health conditions that can exacerbate, aggravate, and irritate them. Many lifestyle irritants contribute to normal fatigue and stress, such as sleep deprivation, poor diet, too much caffeine, and smoking. At the end of this chapter, you'll find a chart I've developed that helps you sort out how your discomforts are connected to your period. Many of you may have solved your "PMS problems" by the end of this chapter.

A Closer Look at Stress

Stress is a chief cause of many of the premenstrual physical ailments. The most important message about this section is that progesterone receptors do not function in the presence of adrenaline, which is the main "stress hormone" that we also make when our blood sugar is low. That is *huge news* that may solve millions of women's PMS problems. (If you look at all the things progesterone regulates in our bodies, shown in Table 8.1, it's easy to see how insufficient progesterone can wreak havoc.) Several studies have linked more severe premenstrual changes to stress. And the studies state what I've been emphasizing all along in this book: Women who have significant life stresses are more likely to experience severe premenstrual changes, which is what the medical community calls "PMS."

Generally, stress is defined as a negative emotional experience associated with biological changes that allow you to adapt to the stress. In response to stress, your adrenal glands pump out "stress hormones" that speed up your body: your heart rate increases and your blood sugar levels increase so that glucose can be diverted to your muscles in case you have to "run." This is known as the "fight or flight" response. These hormones are called the catecholamines, which are broken down into epinephrine (adrenaline), norepinephrine, and dopamine. Katharina Dalton's work has shown that adrenaline prevents progesterone receptors from functioning, which can obviously affect premenstrual changes. So by understanding stress, and making lifestyle changes to lower it, you may be able to dramatically reduce your premenstrual discomforts.

The problem with stress hormones in the 21st century is that the fight or flight response isn't usually necessary, since most of our stress stems from interpersonal situations rather than being chased by a predator. Occasionally, we may want to flee from a bank robber or mugger, but most of us just want to flee from our jobs or our kids! In other words, our stress hormones actually put a physical strain on our bodies and can lower our resistance to disease. Initially, stress hormones stimulate our immune systems. But after the stressful event has passed, stress can suppress the immune system, leaving us open to a wide variety of illnesses and physical symptoms.

Hans Selye, considered the "father" of stress management, defined stress as "wear and tear" on the body. Once we are in a state of stress, the body adapts to the stress by depleting its resources until it becomes exhausted. When the wear and tear on our bodies mounts, we can suffer from stress-related problems:

- Allergies and asthma
- Back pain
- Cardiovascular problems
- Dental and periodontal problems
- Depression

- Emotional outbursts (rage, anger, crying, irritation — seen in recent reports on "air rage" and "road rage")
- Fatigue
- Gastrointestinal problems (digestive disorders, bowel problems, and so on)
- Headaches
- Herpes recurrences (especially in women)
- High blood pressure
- High cholesterol
- Immune suppression (predisposing us to viruses such as colds and flu, infections, autoimmune disorders, and cancer)
- Insomnia
- Loss of appetite and weight loss
- Muscular aches and pains
- Premature aging
- Sexual problems
- Skin problems and rashes

Table 4.1 cross-checks stress-related signs against the physical premenstrual signs (all in alphabetical order). If enough of the problems merge, you need to ask, "Is it stress or PMS"?

As you can see from this lengthy list, stress greatly contributes to ill health and disease. Addictions and substance abuse may fuel many of these problems when we try to relieve our symptoms or self-medicate. Current statistics reveal that 43 percent of all adults suffer from health problems directly caused by stress, while 75 to 90 percent of all visits to primary care physicians are for stress-related complaints or disorders. In the workplace alone, about a million people per day call in sick because of stress, which translates into about 550 million absences per year. Other studies show that roughly 50 percent of all North American workers suffer from "burnout" — a state of mental exhaustion and fatigue caused by stress, while 40 percent of employee turnover is directly caused by stress.

The financial toll of occupational stress to North American industry adds up to about $300 billion annually; this figure was arrived at by factoring in absenteeism, lower productivity, employee turnover, and direct medical, legal, and insurance fees. California employers spend about $1 billion annually for medical and legal fees due to stress, while 90 percent of job stress lawsuits are successful, paying out four times

TABLE 4.1   Stress or PMS?

Unique to Stress	Unique to PMS	Common to Stress and PMS
Dental and periodontal problems	Abdominal bloating (which may also cause weight gain)	Allergies and asthma
Herpes recurrences (especially in women)	Breast swelling and tenderness	Back pain
High blood pressure	Chills, shakiness, and dizziness	Changes in sex drive (either more or less)
High cholesterol	Clumsiness and poor coordination	Depression
Loss of appetite and weight loss	Constipation	Diarrhea
Premature aging	Eye problems	Emotional outbursts (rage, anger, crying, irritation — seen in recent reports on "air rage" and "desk rage")
	Hoarseness	Fatigue
	Increased appetite and weight gain	Gastrointestinal problems (digestive disorders, bowel problems, and so on)
	Nausea	Headaches
	Menopausal-like hot flashes	Heart pounding
	Seizures	Immune-suppression (predisposing us to viruses, such as colds and flu; infections; autoimmune disorders, and cancer)
	Sensitivity to noise	Insomnia
	Sugar and salt cravings	Joint and muscle pain
		Skin problems and rashes

that of other injury claims. Meanwhile, stress management programs grew from a cost of $9.4 billion in 1995 to $11.31 billion in 1999. A more subtle but compelling statistic is this: In 1997 the Japanese word *karoshi,* which means "sudden death from overwork," was found in English dictionaries.

But worse, terrible industry accidents such as oil spills or nuclear reactor accidents, are considered to be caused — 60 to 80 percent of the time — by overstressed workers. Terms such as "office rage" or "desk rage" are emerging, too, as workplace violence escalates.

Types of Stress

Managing your stress is no easy feat, particularly since there are different types of stress: acute stress (which can be episodic) and chronic stress. Acute stress results from a specific situation, such as a sudden, unexpected negative event, or organizing a wedding or planning for a conference. When the event passes, the stress will pass. Acute stress is when you're feeling the pressure of a particular deadline or event. But there is an end to the stress. Acute stress has numerous symptoms: anger or irritability, anxiety, and depression; tension headaches or migraines; back pain, jaw pain, muscular tension; digestive problems; cardiovascular problems; and dizziness.

But acute stress can be what's known as "episodic," meaning that there is one stressful event after another creating a continuous flow of acute stress. Someone who is always taking on too many projects at once is someone who suffers from *episodic* acute stress. Workaholics and those with the so-called "Type A" personality are classic sufferers of episodic acute stress.

I sometimes refer to acute stress as the "good stress" because, often, good things come from this kind of stress, even though it feels "stressful" or bad in the short term. This is the kind of stress that challenges us to stretch ourselves beyond our capabilities, which is what makes us meet deadlines, push the "outside of the envelope," and invent creative solutions to our problems. Examples of events that cause "good" stress include challenging projects, positive life-changing events (moving, changing jobs, or ending unhealthy relationships), and confronting fears, illness, or people who make us feel bad (this is one of those bad in the short term/good in the long term situations). Essentially, whenever a stressful event triggers emotional, intellectual, or spiritual growth, it is a "good stress." It is often not the event as much as it is your *response* to the event that determines whether it is a "good" or "bad" stress. The death of a loved one can sometimes lead to personal growth because we may see something about ourselves we did not see before — new resilience, for example. So even a death can be a "good stress" although we grieve and are sad in the short term.

What I call the "bad stress" is known as chronic stress. Chronic or bad stress results from boredom and stagnation, as well as prolonged negative circumstances. Essentially, when no growth occurs from the stressful event, it is "bad stress." When negative events don't seem to yield anything positive in the long term but more of the *same*, the stress can lead to chronic and debilitating health problems. This is not to say that we can't get sick from good stress, either, but when there is nothing positive from the stress, it has a much more negative effect on our health. Some examples of bad stress include stagnant jobs or relationships, disability from terrible accidents or diseases, long-term unemployment, chronic poverty, racism, or lack of opportunities for change. These kinds of situations can lead to depression, low self-esteem, and a host of physical illnesses.

In addition to acute and chronic stress, there are types of stress that can be defined in even more precise ways:

- Physical stress (physical exertion)

- Chemical stress (when we're exposed to a toxin in our environment, including substance abuse)

- Mental stress (when we take on too much responsibility and begin worrying about all that has to be done)

- Emotional stress (when our feelings stress us out, such as anger, fear, frustration, sadness, betrayal, bereavement)

- Nutritional stress (when we're deficient in certain vitamins or nutrients, overindulged in fat or protein, or experience food allergies)

- Traumatic stress (caused by trauma to the body such as infection, injury, burns, surgery, or extreme temperatures)

- Psycho-spiritual stress (caused by unrest in our personal relationships or belief system, personal life goals, and so on. In general, this is what defines whether we are happy.)

Electronic Stress

Stress management experts have identified electronic stress, or "e-stress," as a new type of stress. For most people, e-mail, voicemail, cell phones, fax machines, pagers, and the other forms of technology that are part of our lives have only lengthened our workdays and given us less time to ourselves. Twenty-five years ago, when you called someone who wasn't home, the phone rang many times and that was it. There was not an onus on the "called" to return your call; the onus was on the caller to call back if she or he needed to get in touch. But with voicemail, the onus is on the called to return the call or, in fact, to answer numerous calls simultaneously, with the advent of Call Waiting. Today, to avoid phone calls, even more technology is required lest we appear to be antisocial by screening our calls. The greater access to communication that technology provides makes our "to do" lists much longer. And if you've made the mistake of subscribing to e-mail discussion groups, you could be bombarded with e-mails — as many hundreds per day. The benefits and burdens of technology increase with handheld organizers, laptops, and so forth. Even watching television has become infinitely more complicated, with complex remotes that not only power the VCR and stereo system, but can rewire your house!

All of this technology translates into "e-stress." Part of e-stress is the learning curve. Learning the new technological toy can wreak havoc on the central nervous system. And the learning, it seems, never ends, as new gadgets are constantly introduced that make the old gadgets obsolete. New versions of e-mail or fax software are also ever problematic.

Another part of e-stress is the lack of privacy. With so many ways to be contacted, there is no safe haven that is communication-free. There is also the problem of being forced to listen to someone else's private life in public places due to overly loud cell-phone conversations. We've all had those moments when we've glared at someone because we really didn't need to know about their mother's friend's colonoscopy! With each new mode of communication comes new responsibilities to reply. Experts call this "multitasking madness."

All the "e" in your life interferes with normal communication. When you're e-mailing with one hand, talking on the phone with the other, and feeling your pager go off in the same instance, how much focused communication can you deliver? The first step in turning down the "e" is looking at all the ways you're plugged in each day. Ask yourself these questions:

- How many phone lines do you have?
- How do you receive the Internet? If it's via cable or dedicated line, you're never "off."
- How many ways can people reach you?
- How many messages do you receive through each mode of communication? Count everything: e-mail to your office, e-mail to your home, phone messages to your cell phone, your office phone, your voice mail, and so on.
- Does e-mail enhance your interpersonal relationships or detract from them? For example, do you find yourself feeling isolated in spite of all the ways you can contact people? Does your life partner spend his or her time at home with you ... or with the computer? Do your children spend quality time at home or do they spend all of their time online, or playing video and computer games? A 2000 Stanford University study on the societal impact of the Internet found that Internet use caused social isolation, confirming the findings of a 1998 study by researchers at Carnegie Mellon University.

The above questions are designed to help you evaluate the impact of the "e" in your life. Reducing e-stress involves redesigning the technology in your life to work *for* you rather than against you. By implementing just one of the following steps, you can help reduce e-stress.

Set Up Unplugged Time.

Make a decision to be unplugged by a certain time of day — such as after 6:00 p.m. and on weekends. You can even indicate your unplugged zone on your outgoing voicemail: "Hi. You've reached Dale at 555-5555. I check my voicemail between 9 and 6 each day. After that time, I cannot be reached." Turn off your computer after 6:00 p.m., too, and do not check e-mail beyond a certain time. You can also set up automatic e-mail responses that tell people you're away, busy, not answering, and so on.

Use Your Cell Phone Only in Cases of Emergency.

Use your cell phone for outgoing emergency calls only for accidents or something unexpected. Don't give out the number to anyone other than very close family members, and don't turn it on unless it's in an emergency situation. If you have voicemail and e-mail, people don't really need to reach you by cell phone. Don't subscribe to a message service on your cell phone, either. That way, no one *can* leave messages.

Limit Your Gadgets.

If you've survived this long without a handheld device, do you *really* need one? In other words, the more stuff you buy, the more you'll use, and the less time you'll have.

Limit Your Surfing Time.

If you're searching for information about a topic on the Internet (such as stress!), you can be there for days. Give yourself a limited amount of time for research, then say (as I do), "I've done the best I can with the time I have."

Limit the Messages You Save.

Try to write down the information as you get it and erase the message. Otherwise, you'll spend too much time listening to (or reading) old messages.

Eliminate Phone Tag.

Avoid phone tag by leaving a specific message with specific instructions for replying: "Hi, George, this is Su Lin. I wanted to set up a meeting this Thursday, at 1:00 p.m., in front of the Coffee Mill. If you can't make it, e-mail me with an alternate time and place. Otherwise, I'll see you Thursday."

Chapters 6 and 7 will show you ways to reduce stress through diet, lifestyle changes, and herbal supplements. What we do to self-medicate for stress, or *self-stimulate* to keep our jobs, can have an enormous impact on premenstrual discomforts, too!

Based on a survey of the general public, men and women report that the following are "top stressors" (listed alphabetically).

- Athletic events
- Attitude toward self
- Demands at the office
- Emotional challenges — personal relationships, fear, anger
- Family changes — marriage, divorce, separation, a new baby
- Health challenges — illness, injury, surgery, chemical exposures
- Job and career challenges
- Life changes — adolescence, aging, pregnancy, menopause
- Loneliness
- Meeting someone new
- Moving
- Personal financial state
- Physical challenges — weather changes, extreme climates
- Promotion, job loss
- Raising children
- Tests in school
- Traffic tickets

Take a Good Look at Your Lifestyle

A number of the following factors can influence your premenstrual discomforts, making them more severe. By modifying some of your lifestyle habits after ovulation, you may be able to dramatically reduce your premenstrual discomforts.

Alcohol

Several studies have confirmed that the amount of alcohol you consume directly impacts the severity of your premenstrual discomforts. For example, women who report severe PMS are typically found to be heavier drinkers in most (but not all) studies that have looked at this link. However, the more stress in your life, the more likely you are to drink, too, which links back to the stress–PMS theory above.

If you tend to drink wine or other alcoholic beverages to unwind after a stressful day, be aware that alcohol can interfere with sleep patterns and is also a depressant. Initially, alcohol may make you tired, and you may think it's a sleeping aid; but it can wake you up later on, making you wide awake at 2:00 a.m. and preventing you from falling back asleep. Naturally, all of this can aggravate premenstrual discomforts, especially irritability, depression, and fatigue.

Women also metabolize alcohol differently than men, so even when a man and woman are the same weight, women will become intoxicated more easily than men — it has to do with fat distribution. The same woman also tolerates alcohol differently at different times in her cycle. She may become more easily intoxicated just before ovulation, which can aggravate premenstrual signs. Women also tend to be invisible drinkers, drinking alone.

Moderate drinking is defined by fewer than 12 drinks per week, when it is not a daily activity. Moderate drinkers do not use alcohol to cope with stress, nor do they plan their recreational activities around alcohol. If you think you're drinking more heavily, keeping a diary of your drinking is useful. Often, just being aware of your alcohol consumption patterns can be enough for you to change your habits.

Alcohol, Blood Sugar, and Weight Gain

Alcohol plays into some specific premenstrual complaints, such as blood sugar stability and the weight gain/bloat problem. Alcohol delivers about 7 calories per gram or 150 calories per drink. Many people think that alcohol is high in sugar and can increase your blood sugar, but this is not so. Alcohol *alone* doesn't increase blood sugar, since alcohol cannot be turned into glucose. It's the sugar *in* that alcoholic beverage that can affect blood sugar levels.

Dry wines that are listed as 0 (meaning no added sugar in Ontario and British Columbia) or "dry" have no sugar. Wine is made by allowing the natural sugar in fruits or fruit juices to ferment. In fermentation, natural sugar is converted into alcohol. A glass of dry red or white wine has calories but no sugar. And unless extra sugar is added to the wine, there's no way that alcohol will change back into sugar, even in your digestive tract. The same thing goes for cognac, brandy, and dry sherry that contain no sugar.

On the other hand, a sweet wine listed as 3 in Ontario or British Columbia, means that it contains 3 grams of sugar per 100 mL or 3.5-oz. portion. Dessert wines or ice wines are really sweet; they contain about 15 percent sugar, or 10 grams of sugar for a 2-oz. serving. Sweet liqueurs are 35 percent sugar.

A glass of dry wine with your meal adds about 100 calories. Half soda water and half wine (a spritzer) contains half the calories. When you cook with wine, the alcohol evaporates, leaving only the flavor.

If you're a beer drinker, you're basically having some corn, barley, and a couple of teaspoons of malt sugar (maltose) when you drink a bottle of beer. The corn and barley ferment into mostly alcohol and some maltose. Calorie-wise, there are about 150 calories per bottle plus 3 teaspoons of malt sugar. A light beer has fewer calories but contains at least 100 calories per bottle. De-alcoholized beer still has sugar and therefore has calories from sugar, too.

The stiffer the drink, the fatter it gets. Hard liquors such as scotch, rye, gin, and rum are made out of cereal grains; vodka, the Russian staple, is made out of potatoes. In this case, the grains ferment into alcohol. Hard liquor averages about 40 percent alcohol, but has no sugar. Nevertheless, you're looking at about 100 calories per small shot glass, so long as you don't add fruit juice, tomato or clamato juice, or sugary soft drinks.

The Glycogen Factor

Glycogen is the stored sugar your liver keeps handy for emergencies. If your blood sugar needs a boost, the liver will tap into its glycogen stores and convert it into glucose. Alcohol in the liver *blocks* this conversion process. So, if you've been exercising and then go out with friends for a few drinks, unless you've eaten something after your exercise, you may need that glycogen. If you drink to the point of feeling tipsy, the alcohol can cut off the glycogen, causing low blood sugar. So if you're going to drink, *eat!* Always have food with your alcohol. Food delays absorption of alcohol into the bloodstream, providing you with carbohydrates and therefore preventing low blood sugar or hypoglycemia.

Activity

Studies show that women who exercise regularly have less severe PMS. This is particularly the case with the emotional signs, as exercise creates endorphins, "feel-good" hormones that act as a natural antidepressant.

By doing just one of the activities on the list in Table 4.2 once or twice a week, you can significantly lower stress, which is a major aggravator of PMS. More intense activities will create endorphins, while less intense activities will help you find more leisure and enjoyment in your life, which also lowers stress.

TABLE 4.2   Activity by Intensity

More Intense	Less Intense
Aerobics	Badminton
Biking	Bowling
Fitness walking	Croquet
Ice skating	Gardening
Jogging	Golf
Jumping rope	Sailing
Race walking	Strolling
Roller skating	Stretching
Running	
Skiing	
Stepping or stair-climbing	
Swimming	
Tennis	
Trampolining	
Weight training	

Caffeine

Lots of studies show that caffeine causes anxiety and sleeplessness, and it is mildly addictive. Caffeine also worsens premenstrual discomforts. Health Canada recommends that you consume no more than 400 to 450 mg of caffeine per day, which is equal to two eight-ounce mugs of gourmet coffee or four cups of instant coffee. Of course, there are many other sources of caffeine, such as soft drinks, chocolate, tea, and so forth. All sources of caffeine should be taken into account along with Health Canada's recommendations.

As well, you should be aware that caffeine is one of the worst aggravators of stress. Caffeine raises your blood pressure and increases the secretion of adrenaline, one of the stress hormones that can "screw up" your progesterone levels. Table 4.3 is a list of how much caffeine some foods contain, with the milligrams of caffeine in brackets.

Smoking

Smoking, or nicotine, can also aggravate stress, which will aggravate premenstrual discomforts. But worse, roughly half a million North Americans die of smoking-related illnesses each year. That's 20 percent of *all* deaths from *all* causes. We already

TABLE 4.3   The Java Chart

Coffee (5-oz./150-mL cup)

Brewed, drip method (60–180)

Brewed, percolator (40–170)

Instant (30–120)

Decaffeinated, brewed (2–5)

Decaffeinated, instant (1–5)

Tea (5-oz./150-mL cup)

Brewed, major brands (20–90)

Brewed, imported brands (25–110)

Iced tea, 12-oz./355-mL glass (67–76)

Instant (25–50)

Other

Caffeine-containing soft drink, 6 oz./180 mL (15–30)

Cocoa beverage, 5 oz./150-mL (2–20)

Chocolate milk, 8 oz./235 mL (2–7)

Milk chocolate, 1-oz./30-mL serving (1–15)

Dark chocolate, semisweet, 1-oz./30-mL serving (5–35)

Baker's chocolate, single square (26)

Chocolate-flavored syrup, 1 serving (4)

know that smoking causes lung cancer. But did you know that smokers are also *twice* as likely to develop heart disease? A single cigarette affects your body within seconds, increasing heart rate, blood pressure, and the demand for oxygen. The greater the demand for oxygen (because of constricted blood vessels and carbon monoxide, a by-product of cigarettes) the greater the risk of heart disease.

Lesser-known long-term effects of smoking include a lowering of HDL, the "good" cholesterol, and damage to the lining of blood vessel walls, which paves the way for arterial plaque formation. In addition to increasing your risk for lung cancer and heart disease, smoking can lead to stroke, peripheral vascular disease, and a host of cancers.

Take a look at some of the things you'll gain by quitting smoking:

- Decreased risk of heart disease
- Decreased risk of cancer (including cancer of the lung, esophagus, mouth, throat, pancreas, kidney, bladder, and cervix)
- Lower heart rate and blood pressure

- Deceased risk of lung disease (bronchitis, emphysema)
- Relaxation of blood vessels
- Improved sense of smell and taste
- Better teeth
- Fewer wrinkles

Many women turn to cigarettes to deal with the demands of stress, as well as for weight control. Studies reveal that people who smoke every day are twice as likely to suffer from depression as people who don't smoke, and depression will, of course, aggravate premenstrual mood swings. That said, mood swings and depression may have nothing to do with smoking and *everything* to do with stressful circumstances; in other words, people under a lot of stress are more likely to suffer from depression or mood swings, and a great deal of those people are likely to smoke to try to calm themselves. Other studies have found that people with depression were three times as likely to be daily smokers. Nicotine may also be a drug we crave to medicate our depressed moods. See Chapter 6 for smoking cessation information.

Weight

Some studies show that women who are overweight are more likely to suffer from more severe premenstrual discomforts. This is because fat cells make estrogen, which can increase the severity of premenstrual hormonal changes. See Chapter 6, "The Diet and Lifestyle Approach, for more information on the weight–PMS connection.

A Closer Look at Fatigue

Fatigue is one of the most common premenstrual complaints. It's important to understand how sick you can feel when you're suffering from just plain old fatigue and stress due to lack of sleep, overwork, and "garden variety" annoyances. The cure is obvious: get more sleep and don't work so hard! Trite advice for such demanding times! In other words, most of us can't afford the cure if we want to keep paying the mortgage or rent.

It's no big secret that women these days are tired and stressed. Most women have multiple roles, juggling career and family pressures. If you're over 40, chances are you're caring for an ailing parent as well as your own children.

There is a difference between feeling normal fatigue, and chronic fatigue. Chronic fatigue is characterized by low energy, lethargy, and flu-like symptoms. This section outlines some of the factors responsible for normal fatigue, which can be remedied by making some lifestyle changes.

Sleep Deprivation

Women who have demanding jobs that require long hours are often sleep deprived, which can have serious health repercussions. Recent research into sleep deprivation has found that it not only depletes the immune system (meaning it depletes you of certain cells needed to destroy viruses and cancerous cells), but it can promote the growth of fat instead of muscle, which may have some interplay with circulating estrogen, because fat cells make estrogen.

Lack of sleep increases levels of the hormone *cortisol*, which is the "stress hormone." As cortisol levels rise, muscle-building human growth hormone and prolactin, a breast-feeding hormone that also helps to protect the immune system, both decrease. Cortisol is released by the adrenal gland in response to stress; it is an "alert" hormone that makes you take action. This is what causes you to be alert in important meetings, close the sale or deal, or suddenly become incredibly articulate with someone on the phone after spending five days with two toddlers without any relief. The hormone will subside in the body as the stressful event passes. Normally during sleep, cortisol levels should decline, while human growth hormone and prolactin should increase. Cortisol declines prior to sleep because it is the body's way of preparing for sleep. Cortisol normally increases in the morning to make you more alert.

There are two types of sleep: rapid eye movement (REM) and non-rapid eye movement. REM sleep is when researchers believe we dream, an important component in mental health. Non-REM sleep is when we are in our deepest sleep, which researchers believe is when various hormones are reset and energy stores are replenished. Right now, we know that roughly 50 percent of people diagnosed with depression (see Chapter 3) get too much REM sleep and not enough deep sleep, which is the "replenishing" sleep.

Energy Drains

Most energy drains come in the form of people. When you're surrounded by people who take energy from you, rather than give you energy in the form of support, the result is fatigue and stress. By doing a serious re-evaluation of your personal relationships, you may be able find more energy. Ask yourself some of the following questions:

- Do you have someone in your life that offers judgment-free emotional support? This is a person who makes you feel positive about yourself rather than a person who points out your flaws or attacks your choices.

- Are there people in your life who drain your energy and reserves? These are people who always seem to be in crisis and suck up large amounts of "free therapy" time from you, but who never seem to be there for you. They can also be people who criticize you and make you feel negative and hopeless instead of positive and optimistic.

- Do you have unresolved conflicts with family members or friends? These unresolved feelings can drain your energy and focus, as we tend to obsess over the conflict over and over again.

- Do you feel your friends are more "acquaintances" and that you lack truly intimate friendships?

- Are you in a romantic or sexual relationship that you need to end, but have been avoiding doing so?

- Are you in a relationship that compromises your values?

- Is there a phone call you need to make or some other obligation that you are avoiding that is causing you fatigue, stress, and anxiety?

- Is there someone in your life who continuously breaks commitments or plans, with whom you are constantly rescheduling?

Energy drains can also come from unmet needs in your home environment. Do you have broken appliances, car repairs that haven't been done, a wardrobe you hate, cluttered closets and rooms, or even ugly surroundings? Living in a home that is not decorated in a way that pleases you makes you feel as though you don't want to be there. Plants, paint, covers for ugly furniture, and a few things on the wall often make the difference between barren and dank surroundings and cozy. See Chapter 6, "The Diet and Lifestyle Approach," for more on the "little things" in life that make huge differences to your stress quotient.

Finally, energy drains come from procrastinating and overbooking yourself. We procrastinate over things we really don't want to do — such as taxes. We overbook ourselves when we're afraid of saying no. Every article and book on stress management has these trite three words of advice: "Just say no." The problem is, few people will ever say it. Instead of "No," try: "Let me check my schedule and see if I'm already committed." Then, "Sorry, looks like I'm committed elsewhere," or if it's a task, "I've got a deadline on that date for something of equal importance."

Simply doing too much, and expecting too much from ourselves, drains our energy. At home, consider hiring someone to

- Clean your house or apartment
- De-clutter your home by going through closets, filing things, and so on
- Organize your tax receipts
- Garden and/or take care of your lawn

Chronic Fatigue

Chronic fatigue is not the same thing as normal fatigue. It is a continuing fatigue, accompanied by other symptoms of malaise that no amount of sleep seems to solve. Seventy percent of all people who suffer from chronic fatigue are women under the age of 45. Many of them may be misdiagnosed with "PMS" or depression. Chronic fatigue syndrome (CFS) has been around longer than you might think. In 1843, for example, a curious condition called "fibrositis" was described by doctors, which was characterized by similar symptoms now seen in *fibromyalgia* (chronic muscle and joint aches and pains) and *chronic fatigue syndrome* (symptoms of fibromyalgia, accompanied by flu-like symptoms and extreme fatigue). The term "rheumatism," an outdated label, was frequently used as well to describe various aches and pains with no specific or identifiable origin.

In the late 1970s and early 1980s, a mysterious virus, known as the Epstein-Barr virus, was being diagnosed in thousands of young, upwardly mobile professionals — who at the time were known as "yuppies." People were calling this condition the "yuppie flu," the "yuppie virus," "yuppie syndrome," and "burn-out" syndrome. Many medical professionals were stumped by it, and many disregarded it as a phantom illness or a psychosomatic illness. Because so many women were dismissed by their doctors as hypochondriacs, or were not believed to be ill or fatigued, the physical symptoms triggered self-doubts, and feelings of low self-esteem, self-loathing, and so on, which often triggered depression. But even with the most sensitive medical attention, depression seems to go hand in hand with CFS simply because the disorder leaves so many sufferers at home in bed, isolated from the active lifestyle they once had. In other words, some believe that in the case of CFS, depression is a normal response to "feeling like shit" every day of your life!

Take a look at the established symptom criteria for CFS on the next page. In the early 1980s, two physicians in Nevada, who treated a number of patients who shared this curious condition (after a nasty winter flu had hit the region), identified it as "chronic fatigue syndrome." This label, perhaps the most accurate, is the one that has stuck.

But there are some other names for CFS, such as the U.K. label, myalgic encephalomyelitis (ME), as well as post-viral fatigue syndrome. CFS is also known as chronic fatigue immune deficiency syndrome (CFIDS), because it's now believed that CFS sufferers are immune-suppressed, although this is still in debate. But for the purposes of this chapter, I'll refer to the simpler label that seems to tell it like it is: chronic fatigue syndrome.

The Symptoms of CFS

The term chronic fatigue syndrome refers to a *collection* of ill-health symptoms (not just one or two), the most identifiable of which are fatigue and flu-like aches and pains.

It wasn't until 1994 that an official definition of CFS was actually published in the Annals of Internal Medicine. The Centers for Disease Control (CDC) have since published official symptoms of CFS, too. Although many physicians feel the following list of symptoms is limiting and requires some expansion for accuracy, as of this writing, the official defining symptoms of CFS include the following:

1. An unexplained fatigue that is "new." In other words, you've previously felt fine, and have only noticed in the last six months or so that you're always fatigued, no matter how much rest you get. The fatigue is also debilitating for you; you're not as productive at work, and it interferes with normal activities that may be social, personal, or academic. You've also noticed poor memory or concentration, which affects your activities and performance, too.

2. In addition to this fatigue, you have four or more of the following symptoms, which have persisted for at least six months:

   - Sore throat

   - Mild or low-grade fever

   - Tenderness in the neck and underarm area (these are where you have lymph nodes, which may be swollen, causing tenderness)

   - Muscle pain (called myalgia)

   - Pain along the nerve of a joint, without redness or swelling

   - A strange and new kind of headache you've never suffered from before

   - Waking up unrefreshed (a sign of insufficient amounts of non-REM sleep, as discussed earlier in this chapter)

- Feeling tired, weak, and generally unwell for a good 24 hours after you've had even moderate exercise

3. Poor exercise tolerance.

Some CFS experts feel that "poor exercise tolerance," (meaning that even modest exercise is followed by such exhaustion and malaise that you can't tolerate it) is perhaps the hallmark symptom of CFS. Research into CFS has uncovered that there is indeed a biological reason for this that has to do with a deficient flow of oxygen and energy to your cells during exercise. Normally, oxygen increases in our bodies with exercise; in CFS sufferers, the opposite has been found: oxygen seems to decrease with exercise, which may explain a lot! Without oxygen during exercise, various "poisons" (accumulated substances we produce naturally, such as lactic acid, magnesium, etc.) can build up and reduce the efficiency of our tissues and organs. Why this is happening remains to be discovered, while the issue of whether this is happening at all still needs to be confirmed and further documented, according to many other scientists.

Fibromyalgia versus CFS

Fibromyalgia is a soft-tissue disorder that causes you to hurt all over — all the time. The condition appears to be triggered and/or aggravated by stress. If you notice fatigue and general aches and pains, this suggests CFS. If you notice *primarily* joint and muscle pains, *accompanied* by fatigue, this suggests fibromyalgia.

Fibromyalgia is considered by some to be an offshoot of arthritis, and a misdiagnosis of rheumatoid arthritis is not unusual. Headaches, morning stiffness, and an intolerance to cold, damp weather are common complaints with fibromyalgia. It's also common to suffer from irritable bowel syndrome or bladder problems with this disorder.

Causes of CFS

There is no official, known cause of CFS. But there are several theories. One theory suggests that viral agents are infecting the population (the book *Osler's Web* suggests this is the case, and further suggests there is an active government cover-up of such viruses). Another theory is that airborne environmental toxins and poisons impact the immune system.

Some CFS sufferers have an impaired immune system, similar to what happens with HIV infection. This suggests there *may* be some viral agent(s) at work. But other CFS sufferers have an overactive immune system, suggesting that CFS may be an autoimmune condition, meaning that your immune system manufactures antibodies that attack your body's own tissues. Autoimmune diseases are triggered by stress. The pain and inflammation many CFS sufferers report is more likely due to an overactive immune system; the flu-like malaise and fatigue is more likely due to an underactive immune system. This is why CFS remains a mystery to researchers. However, when a body is poisoned by environmental toxins, it's possible that different toxins can trigger different reactions by the immune system, which may explain the paradox. Gulf War Syndrome, for example, is characterized by a wide array of symptoms. Different bodies may react differently to the same toxin, too.

Stress appears to be a major trigger of CFS, as well. When we are under stress, our bodies produce the hormone adrenaline, which increases our heart rate, blood flow, blood pressure, and so on. Adrenaline may aggravate the inflammation and pain many CFS and fibromyalgia sufferers experience.

Some experts who treat CFS and fibromyalgia believe that a lack of non-REM sleep may be a factor in this disorder. Some experts have gone on record to say that chronic fatigue syndrome is really a sleep-related disorder. One Canadian study deliberately deprived a group of medical students of non-REM sleep over a period of several nights. Within the next few days, each of the study participants developed symptoms of CFS and/or fibromyalgia.

Treatments

Most experts agree that CFS is an environmental illness, triggered by stress. Diet and lifestyle modification appear to be effective ways to treat CFS, as certain "trigger foods" — foods that typically trigger allergies or fungal infections with the fungus *Candida albicans* (such as processed foods and foods high in sugar or yeast) are eliminated and replaced with more nutritious vitamin-packed foods that are organic. Candida is a parasite that normally inhabits our digestive tract. This parasite can overgrow and spread to other places in the body, damaging the immune system. Since so many CFS sufferers have candida, adjusting the diet is a logical first step.

Often a move to a cleaner environment is useful (changing jobs or telecommuting if you believe you're being exposed to workplace toxins; moving from an urban center to a suburb or rural area).

"Downshifting" — a term coined to describe simplifying lifestyles, shedding the urban "noise and toys" — often works wonders to shed some stress, which can often improve CFS. This may involve moving to a smaller place with a lower monthly payment, leaving a job, buying that farm you've always wanted, or blowing your "retirement money" and taking a long trip. (This was known in the 1960s as "dropping out.")

CFS experts and fellow sufferers caution you about taking antidepressants — often the first thing a medical doctor will prescribe. Since antidepressants have many side effects that can aggravate CFS symptoms, they are reportedly not the best solution as a "first line" treatment for CFS. The general advice is to try cleaning up your diet and lifestyle first and see whether your symptoms improve. Symptoms of depression in CFS often resolve when you start to feel a little better physically and get out of the house!

Numerous alternative therapies are reported to work with CFS. Review my list of CFS resources at the back of this book. Many of these organizations have websites, monthly newsletters with the "latest" treatment trends, and so on. I hesitate, as of this writing, to recommend much of what I came across in my research because it is simply not substantiated yet. But like so many herbs and alternative therapies, ranging from glucosamine sulphate (for arthritis) to St. John's wort, just because they're not proven in traditional scientific studies doesn't mean they don't work. Time will tell, as well as word of mouth. To date, however, diet modification is the most effective treatment CFS experts recommend, along with cognitive therapy, which is a type of counseling that helps you to "shift" your thinking or focus.

Could PMS Be a Blood Sugar Problem?

The most important thing to remember about this section is this: progesterone receptors do not work when your blood sugar is low. (Refer to Table 8.1 to see what progesterone does in the body.) The connection between progesterone and blood sugar is *huge news*, and may account for millions of women's PMS problems.

Understanding blood sugar is pretty complicated. Estrogen influences your blood sugar levels and insulin requirements. There is also evidence that estrogen-containing products can even trigger insulin resistance in women who have a family history or genetic predisposition to Type 2 diabetes (which used to be called adult onset diabetes, a completely different disease from Type 1 diabetes, which used to be called juvenile diabetes). Estrogen usually *raises* blood sugar levels. This is why estrogen-containing medications, such as oral contraceptives or hormone replacement therapy after menopause, were once considered "no-no's" for women with diabetes. It is also why "diabetes" is still labeled a *contraindication* (meaning a condition that is not compatible with a given therapy or medication) for many estrogen-containing products.

But what women are *not* told by their doctors is that when they take any synthetic estrogen or progestin (the synthetic version of progesterone) they can frequently develop hypoglycemia, meaning "low blood sugar," which can become badly aggravated premenstrually due to a natural rise in insulin levels after ovulation. A rise in insulin and a dip in blood sugar account for several severe premenstrual physical changes, including changes in appetite and cravings.

Even if you're not taking artificial estrogen products, when estrogen levels are naturally high during the premenstrual part of your cycle, your body may be more resistant to its own insulin, and this may be a major reason for the sugar cravings in particular. *Insulin increases our appetite.* Women with diabetes find that their blood sugar levels will be high for about three to five days before, during, or after their periods. But blood sugar levels may be higher in all women premenstrually due to the influences of estrogen. And high blood sugar can create very severe premenstrual changes. On top of blood sugar fluctuations, food cravings are caused by an increase in progesterone at this time in your cycle, which affects all women equally — regardless of whether they have diabetes.

Dr. Katharina Dalton developed the "Three Hourly Starch Diet" as she recognized the relationship between carbohydrates and severe mood swings and other premenstrual changes. I discuss this diet, as well as other approaches to meal planning in Chapter 6, "The Diet and Exercise Approach."

Signs of Type 2 Diabetes

Type 2 diabetes is a genetic disease that is triggered by environmental factors, such as obesity or a sedentary lifestyle. Women who developed gestational diabetes during a pregnancy are also more likely to develop Type 2 diabetes. Generally, Type 2 diabetes is more common in women who are overweight and is especially on the rise in women of color and rampant in Native women.

Type 2 diabetes is a disease of insulin resistance rather than no insulin. The disease causes your body to overproduce insulin. Too much insulin leads to a decrease in insulin-receptor sites, small "keyholes" on the surface of your insulin-producing cells, into which insulin (the "key") fits. Sometimes there are simply not enough receptor sites; other times, something is wrong with the connection or link between the key and keyhole. The end result is that your body's cells are not responding to the insulin you are making. If you have any of the symptoms listed below, request to be screened for Type 2 diabetes, which is done through a blood glucose test.

The following are common symptoms of Type 2 diabetes:

- Weight gain (when you're not using your insulin properly, you may suffer from excess insulin, which can increase your appetite — this is a classic Type 2 symptom)

- Blurred vision or any change in sight (often there is a feeling that your prescription eyewear is "weak")

- Drowsiness or *extreme* fatigue at times when you shouldn't be drowsy or tired

- Frequent infections that are slow to heal (women should be on alert for recurring vaginal yeast infections or vaginitis, which means vaginal inflammation, characterized by itching and/or foul-smelling discharge)

- Tingling or numbness in the hands and feet

- Gum disease (high blood sugar affects the blood vessels in your mouth, causing inflamed gums; the sugar content can get into your saliva, causing cavities in your teeth.)

Diabetes experts point out that the following may also be signs of Type 2 diabetes:

- Irregular periods, such as changes in cycle length or flow

- Depression, which could be a symptom of either low or high blood sugar

- Headaches (from hypoglycemia)

- Insomnia and/or nightmares (from hypoglycemia)

- Spots on the shin (known as *Necrobiosis lipoidica diabeticorum*)

- Decaying toenails

- Muscle pains or aches after exercise (high blood sugar can cause lactic acid to build up, which can cause pain that prevents you from continuing exercise)

Signs of Hypoglycemia

A normal blood sugar reading before eating is 4 to 6 millimoles per liter (mmol/l). Technically, any blood sugar reading below 3.5 mmol/l is considered too low, but women can have signs of hypoglycemia with blood sugar readings that doctors tell them are "normal." The way to test it is to drink some juice as you feel the symptoms coming on to see if it alleviates the symptoms. If it does, your PMS problems may be a blood sugar problem instead.

A hypoglycemic episode is characterized by two stages: the warning stage and what I call the *actual* hypoglycemic episode. The warning stage occurs when your blood sugar levels *begin* to drop, and can occur as early as a blood sugar reading of 6 mmol/l, in people with typically higher than normal blood sugar levels. When your blood sugar drops to the 3.5 mmol/l range, you are *officially* hypoglycemic.

During the warning stage, your body responds by piping adrenaline into your bloodstream. This causes symptoms such as trembling, irritability, hunger, and weakness (see the complete list of warning symptoms below). The irritability can be similar to the ranting of someone who is drunk, while the weakness and shakiness can lead to the lack of coordination seen in someone who is drunk. Your liver will also release any glucose it has stored for you; but if it doesn't have enough glucose to get you back to normal, there won't be enough glucose for your brain to function normally and you will feel confused, irritable, or aggressive.

If you are diabetic, hypoglycemia can be particularly serious and can cause you to lose consciousness and perhaps undergo a seizure. Not everyone experiences the same warning symptoms, but here is a complete list:

- Pounding, racing heart
- Breathing fast
- Skin turning white
- Sweating (cold sweat in big drops)
- Trembling, tremors, or shaking
- Goose bumps or pale, cool skin
- Extreme hunger pangs
- Light-headedness (feeling dizzy or that the room is spinning)
- Nervousness, extreme irritability, or a sudden mood change
- Confusion
- Feeling weak or faint
- Headache
- Vision changes (seeing double or blurry vision)

How to Deal with an Attack

If you feel you are in the throes of a "low," the best way to get your levels back up to normal is to ingest simple sugar; that is, sugar that gets into your bloodstream fast. Half a cup of any fruit juice or one-third of a can of a sugary soft drink is a good source of simple sugar. Artificially sweetened soft drinks are useless. *It must have real sugar.* If you don't have fruit juice or soft drinks handy, here are some other sources high in simple sugar:

- Two to three tablets of commercial dextrose, sold in pharmacies (you can keep this on hand)
- Three to five hard candies (that's equal to about six Life Savers)

TABLE 4.4   Blood Sugar or PMS?

Unique to Blood Sugar Problems	Unique to PMS	Common to Blood Sugar Problems and PMS
Decaying toenails	Abdominal bloating	Clumsiness and poor coordination
Frequent infections (especially yeast infections)	Acne or other skin eruptions	Depression
Gum disease	Asthma	Drowsiness
Spots on the shin (known as *Necrobiosis lipoidica diabeticorum*)	Backache	Eye problems
	Breast swelling and tenderness	Fatigue
Tingling or numbness in the hands and feet	Changes in sex drive (either more or less)	Food cravings
	Chills	Headaches
	Constipation or diarrhea	Heart pounding
	Hoarseness	Insomnia and/or nightmares
	Menopausal-like hot flashes	Irregular periods
	Nausea	Joint and muscle pain
	Seizures	Shakiness and dizziness
	Sensitivity to noise	Weight gain and appetite increase

- Two teaspoons of white or brown sugar (or two sugar cubes)
- One tablespoon of honey

Table 4.4 compares the symptoms of blood sugar problems with PMS.

Could PMS Be a Thyroid Problem?

When factors such as stress, low blood sugar, or taking synthetic estrogen and progestin block your progesterone receptors, depriving your body of adequate amounts of progesterone, this can also affect how much thyroid hormone goes to your cells (the role of progesterone is explained in Table 8.1). Thyroid is a key hormone we need to function. When we are deprived of it, we become *hypothyroid,* which technically means your thyroid is underactive. It may be that your thyroid is normal but your body's cells may not be receiving the hormone it's making in adequate amounts due to "screwed up" levels of progesterone. This problem can aggravate premenstrual discomforts. The way to solve the problem is to investigate natural progesterone therapy. Or you can supplement your thyroid hormone with thyroid hormone replacement. Other causes of hypothyroidism include inflammation of the thyroid gland, postpartum thyroid inflammation, or as a result of treatment for hyperthyroidism (an overactive thyroid gland — see further on) or thyroid cancer.

Signs of Hypothyroidism

When you're hypothyroid, everything slows down — including your body temperature. Table 4.5 describes hypothyroidism, and Table 4.6 compares the symptoms of hypothyroidism to those of PMS.

TABLE 4.5   Hypothyroidism At a Glance

Women are five times more likely to experience hypothyroidism than men. Here's a quick checklist of symptoms.

What You May Notice (listed alphabetically)

☐ Changes in skin pigmentation	☐ Headaches
☐ Chest pain after physical activity	☐ Irregular periods or infertility
☐ Constipation	☐ Loss of interest in sex
☐ Depression	☐ Muscle spasms
☐ Difficult-to-manage hair, brittle nails	☐ Problems focusing
☐ Difficulty concentrating	☐ Shortness of breath
☐ Extreme tiredness and slowness	☐ Slow healing
☐ Eyelids that feel "sticky"	☐ Tingling in hands and feet
☐ Feeling cold	☐ Weakness and muscular aches and pains
☐ Frequent infections	☐ Weight gain

What Others May Say

☐ "You look pale"

☐ "Your face is puffy"

☐ "Your eyes are swollen"

☐ "Your hair looks/feels coarse," or "Are you losing hair?"

☐ "Your voice is husky"

☐ "You snore!"

☐ "You used to LOVE doing X or Y — why aren't you interested anymore?"

☐ "Did you HEAR what I said?" (meaning that you can't hear well)

What Your Doctor Should Watch For (listed alphabetically)

☐ Delayed reflexes

TABLE 4.5   Hypothyroidism At a Glance (continued)

What Your Doctor Should Watch For (listed alphabetically)

☐ Goiter (enlarged thyroid)

☐ Milk leaking from breasts (when you're not breast-feeding)

☐ Muscle weakness

☐ Slowed pulse

☐ Soft abdomen

☐ Tingling or numbness in the hands (sign of carpal tunnel syndrome)

Source: Adapted from Patsy Westcott, *Thyroid Problems: A Practical Guide To Symptoms and Treatment*, 35.

TABLE 4.6   Hypothyroidism or PMS?

Unique to Hypothyroidism	Unique to PMS	Common to Hypothyroidism and PMS
Changes in skin pigmentation	Asthma	Abdominal bloating
Chest pain after physical activity	Backache	Acne or other skin eruptions
Dry, coarse skin	Breast swelling and tenderness	Brittle fingernails
Dry, brittle hair	Changes in sex drive (either more or less)	Clumsiness and poor coordination
Enlarged thyroid gland		
Frequent infections	Chills	Constipation
Heavier periods	Diarrhea	Depression
High cholesterol	Fatigue	Dizziness
Hives	Heart pounding	Eye problems
Numbness	Increased appetite	Feeling cold
Shortness of breath	Insomnia	Headaches
Slow healing	Menopausal-like hot flashes	Hoarseness
Slow heartbeat	Nausea	Irregular periods or infertility
Tingling in hands and feet	Seizures	Joint and muscle pain
	Sensitivity to noise	Loss of interest in sex
	Sugar and salt cravings	Muscle spasms
		Poor memory and concentration
		Ringing in the ears
		Shakiness

TABLE 4.7 Hyperthyroidism At a Glance

Nine out of 10 hyperthyroid people are women. Here's a quick checklist of hyperthyroid symptoms.

What You May Notice (listed alphabetically)

- ☐ Anxiety and irritability
- ☐ Changes in menstrual cycle, such as no periods, longer or shorter cycle
- ☐ Dry, thin skin that turns red easily
- ☐ Enlarged thyroid
- ☐ Eye problems or irritations
- ☐ Feeling hot all the time
- ☐ Hair loss
- ☐ Increased appetite
- ☐ Increased sex drive
- ☐ Increased sweating
- ☐ Insomnia
- ☐ Muscle weakness
- ☐ Palpitations
- ☐ Staring eyes
- ☐ Warm, moist palms
- ☐ Weight loss

What Others May Say

- ☐ "You're moody"
- ☐ "You're so talkative lately!"
- ☐ "You seem agitated"
- ☐ "Your neck looks swollen"
- ☐ "Why are you staring like that?" (i.e., your eyes have a "staring" look)
- ☐ "You've lost weight"
- ☐ "You're shaking"

What Your Doctor Should Look For (listed alphabetically)

- ☐ Fast pulse
- ☐ Irregular heartbeat (atrial fibrillation)
- ☐ Low blood pressure
- ☐ Quick reflexes
- ☐ Tremor

Source: Adapted from Patsy Westcott, *Thyroid Problems: A Practical Guide To Symptoms and Treatment*, 45.

Testing Your Thyroid Function

Testing for hypothyroidism is done through a simple blood test called the TSH test. A normal TSH reading ranges from 0.5–5. A reading greater than 5 suggests that you're hypothyroid, while a reading less than 5 suggests that you're hyperthyroid (meaning that your gland is overactive). The "norms" for a healthy body are often based on a healthy white male body — one that is not of female or of a different ethnic origin. This has to do with medical research guidelines that were designed to protect women's reproductive organs, which at the same time kept them out of clinical trials. So keep that in mind when you go for any medical test and are told you are "normal" when you do not feel that you're functioning normally for you. There are other tests that can confirm or help shed light on whether you are hypothyroid. For more about thyroid testing, see *The Thyroid Sourcebook for Women* or *The Thyroid Sourcebook,* 4th edition.

TABLE 4.8   Hyperthyroidism or PMS?

Unique to Hyperthyroidism	Unique to PMS	Common to Hyperthyroidism and PMS
Dry, thin skin that turns red easily	Acne or other skin eruptions	Anxiety and irritability
Enlarged thyroid	Abdominal bloating	Changes in menstrual cycle, such as no periods, longer or shorter cycle
Hair loss	Asthma	Clumsiness and poor coordination
Muscle weakness	Backache	Diarrhea
Warm, moist palms	Breast swelling and tenderness	Dizziness
Weight loss	Chills	Eye problems or irritations
	Constipation	Feeling hot
	Depression	Heart pounding
	Fatigue	Increased appetite
	Headaches	Increased sex drive
	Hoarseness	Increased sweating
	Joint and muscle pain	Insomnia
	Loss of interest in sex	Menopausal-like hot flashes
	Nausea	Shakiness
	Poor memory and concentration	Sugar and salt cravings
	Ringing in the ears	
	Seizures	
	Sensitivity to noise	

What about Hyperthyroidism?

Hyperthyroidism is usually caused by an autoimmune disorder known as Graves' disease. It can also occur if you are being overmedicated with thyroid hormone supplements, which is the treatment for hypothyroidism. The symptoms of hyperthyroidism can also badly aggravate PMS. Table 4.7 describes the signs of hyperthyroidism, and Table 4.8 compares the signs of hyperthyroidism to those of PMS.

Charting Physical Premenstrual Signs

Use the chart on the following page to help you determine when in your cycle your physical changes begin and end, "peak and valley." Remember that day 1 of your cycle is the first day of bleeding, or day 1 of your period.

My Physical Cycle Chart

Cycle Day: **Calendar Date:**

Check the boxes to the left that represent the feeling, perception, or experience you have today. Circle the number on the right to rate the degree to which you feel/perceive/experience these things. 10 means "very severe" and 1 means "very mild."

	Very mild							**Very severe**		
[ ] Acne or other skin eruptions	1	2	3	4	5	6	7	8	9	10
[ ] Asthma	1	2	3	4	5	6	7	8	9	10
[ ] Backache	1	2	3	4	5	6	7	8	9	10
[ ] Bloating	1	2	3	4	5	6	7	8	9	10
[ ] Breast swelling and tenderness	1	2	3	4	5	6	7	8	9	10
[ ] Changes in sex drive	1	2	3	4	5	6	7	8	9	10
[ ] Chills	1	2	3	4	5	6	7	8	9	10
[ ] Clumsiness and poor coordination	1	2	3	4	5	6	7	8	9	10
[ ] Constipation	1	2	3	4	5	6	7	8	9	10
[ ] Diarrhea	1	2	3	4	5	6	7	8	9	10
[ ] Dizziness	1	2	3	4	5	6	7	8	9	10
[ ] Eye problems	1	2	3	4	5	6	7	8	9	10
[ ] Fatigue	1	2	3	4	5	6	7	8	9	10
[ ] Increased appetite	1	2	3	4	5	6	7	8	9	10
[ ] Headaches	1	2	3	4	5	6	7	8	9	10
[ ] Heart pounding	1	2	3	4	5	6	7	8	9	10
[ ] Hoarseness	1	2	3	4	5	6	7	8	9	10
[ ] Insomnia	1	2	3	4	5	6	7	8	9	10

		Very mild								Very severe	
[ ] Joint and muscle pain		1	2	3	4	5	6	7	8	9	10
[ ] Menopausal-like hot flashes		1	2	3	4	5	6	7	8	9	10
[ ] Nausea		1	2	3	4	5	6	7	8	9	10
[ ] Salt cravings		1	2	3	4	5	6	7	8	9	10
[ ] Sensitivity to noise		1	2	3	4	5	6	7	8	9	10
[ ] Seizures		1	2	3	4	5	6	7	8	9	10
[ ] Shakiness		1	2	3	4	5	6	7	8	9	10
[ ] Sugar cravings		1	2	3	4	5	6	7	8	9	10
[ ] Weight gain		1	2	3	4	5	6	7	8	9	10

List any medications you're on today.

Aspirin and Tylenol count! List all prescription and over-the-counter medications you're taking.

_____

_____

_____

List any herbal or vitamin supplements you're taking.

_____

_____

_____

What did you eat or drink today?

List your meals and snacks and times you ate them.

_____

_____

_____

Special circumstances

Did anything out of the ordinary occur today? If so, explain.

_____

_____

_____

Moon cycle

Take note of the moon's position so you can chart your physical changes in accordance with moon changes. Remember, menstrual cycle means "moon cycle." Chart any eclipses and so on.

_____

_____

_____

Physical Cycle Chart, Copyright © M. Sara Rosenthal, 2001.

5

FINDING A "PMS DOCTOR"

Just because someone is a doctor, it doesn't mean that she or he is a moral person, a caring person, a nice person, a wise person, or even an especially smart person. In Canada, it often means she or he was good in chemistry, math, and memorizing — the only qualities you really need to get into medical school these days. If you were to look at what doctors actually learn in medical school, you'll find a number of things completely absent from the curriculum: virtually no training in nutrition; no training in herbal medicine or alternative healing systems, which are now so basic to primary care; no training in mind/body medicine; and no formal training in clinical or research ethics. Women who go through medical school are frequently harassed and put down by their teachers, and there are numerous published articles by female doctors who are now "coming out" about their abusive training experiences.

An interest in humanities (such as history and philosophy), good communication skills, or even good listening skills — qualities one might like to see in a doctor from time to time — are just not essential to their training. But when it comes to healing women, all of these "non-essentials" *are absolutely essential*!

A good doctor is one who listens, who cares, and who has an interest in looking at the woman holistically in a mind-body-lifestyle approach. That's the only thing you need to find in a "PMS doctor." In fact, when it comes to remedying your premenstrual discomforts and mood changes, a good old-fashioned grandmother will probably do you more good than the country's top psychiatrist or endocrinologist because, chances are, your discomforts are related to other things going on in your life besides your hormones or serotonin levels. Treating your parts, and not your whole, does not make a good women's physician.

In Canada, doctors are scarce; good doctors are even scarcer. So instead of focusing on finding a good doctor, focus on being a good consumer of medical services by knowing your rights and your options. For example, you have to arm yourself with the right questions — and sometimes the right answers — to stave off instant antidepressant prescriptions. You have to know what "informed consent" actually means, and get full disclosure on drugs you're prescribed or any other treatment being suggested. By the end of this chapter, you'll know more about treating PMS than most doctors. And that will allow you to find the right PMS doctor — because you'll know "what's right" and what's not.

How Doctors Approach PMS

At one time, women's premenstrual physical discomforts and mood swings were dismissed by doctors, and finding the right "PMS doctor" meant finding a doctor who validated that something real and physiological was going on rather than telling the woman that all of her physical and emotional changes were "in her head." This is a common experience in women's health. Women are told to "buzz off" by doctors when they report symptoms of heart attack (we now know that heart attack symptoms manifest completely differently in women), thyroid problems, chronic fatigue syndrome, and a range of other problems.

By the 1970s and early 1980s, PMS was considered by most doctors to be a hormonal disease that required treatment with synthetic hormones. A lot of this approach was based on the pioneering work of Dr. Katharina Dalton, whom I discuss in Chapter 1, "PMS Is Not a Disease." Dalton was the first doctor to call PMS "premenstrual syndrome" and one of the first doctors to call PMS a "hormonal disease." She still insists that the only good way to treat "true PMS" (which means all your bodily changes vanish when you get your period and remain "gone" until after you ovulate) is through *natural* progesterone, since the synthetic stuff (called progestin) does not bind to the progesterone receptors properly, causing more problems than it supposedly solves. Natural progesterone therapy is a good option for you to consider when you've ruled out other underlying causes for your premenstrual discomforts and mood changes (as I describe in Chapters 3 and 4), and when nutritional and herbal approaches fail.

Dalton was the first doctor to validate that PMS is a physical phenomenon. That approach hasn't changed. But feminist critics of women's health care are disturbed by Dalton's belief that PMS is a "hormonal disease." Dalton's own research, in fact, tells us that the following interferes with the body's ability to send enough progesterone to our molecules: low blood sugar (which can be solved by better eating habits), stress (which can be solved by diet and lifestyle changes), and low thyroid hormone (see Chapter 4).

Where feminists, natural progesterone promoters such as Dalton, and health care practitioners with holistic approaches to PMS reach consensus is the belief that PMS is not a psychiatric problem, and antidepressants are not a solution. Psychiatrists got in the game because of all of the emotional changes women experience, and, as Dalton says in her book *Once A Month*, they "hijacked PMS" as their own disease, which they maintain, has "furthered" the cause for women because it allows women to use PMS as a defense in litigation cases, employment disputes, absenteeism, and so on.

Psychiatrists and PMS

Before you see a psychiatrist for PMS, it's useful to have some background on the social history of women, their moods and behaviors, and psychiatric treatment.

The first European "madhouses," as they were called, were nothing short of prisons for unwanted wives and daughters. As early as the 16th century, wives were thrown into madhouses or royal towers by their husbands as punishment for not conforming or "behaving." Soon, "private madhouses" came into vogue, which were for-profit institutions designed as drop-off centers for rich husbands to dump their wives. The practice became so widespread that Daniel Defoe criticized it 1687, calling attention to the "vile practice now so much in vogue among the better sort, as they are called, but the worst sort, in fact, namely the sending of their wives to madhouses at every whim or dislike" (Chesler, 1971: 33–34).

By the 17th century, prostitutes, unmarried pregnant women, poor women, and young girls joined wives in the first mental asylum in France, called the Salpetriere. Women continued to populate mental asylums throughout the 19th century. Until the 1970s, the majority of women in mental hospitals were committed involuntarily, or while they were in a coma following an unsuccessful suicide attempt.

One of the most famous cases of involuntary confinement involved Elizabeth Packard, whose husband committed her to an asylum in 1860 because she dared to question religion. Elizabeth was kidnapped by her husband, who then withheld her children, income (from her inheritance), clothes, books, and so on. Packard began a diary of asylum events (or, rather, horrors), and never referred to it as a hospital but always as a prison. It is Packard who first compared institutional psychiatry to the Inquisition. Many feminist writers observe that the players in the drama of mental hospital "scenes" mimic the witchcraft trials. The male doctors star as the "Inquisitors"; a subservient female nurse stars as the "Handmaiden," while a female patient stars as a "Witch," possessed by unhappiness, powerlessness, and dependence. These images still pervade mental health. In a 1998 article on depression in a women's health magazine, the "visual" accompanying the article was that of a woman lying down on a hospital bed with wires attached to her head and a plastic device inside her mouth. Around her hovered scientific-looking male doctors, with beards and glasses. The article discussed brain research and the differences between male and female brain responses to cortisol, a hormone produced while under stress (see Chapter 4, "The Physical Premenstrual Signs").

According to Phyllis Chesler's research, by the 20th century, many male psychiatrists were acting as agents for husbands unhappy with their wives. This differed from the 17th century in that the husbands now appeared to be innocent bystanders while the psychiatrists recommended institutionalization. By 1964, the number of U.S. women seeking psychiatric services climbed to unprecedented rates, and adult female patients exceeded the number of adult male patients.

As of 1992, women accounted for roughly two-thirds of psychiatric consumers; 84 percent of all psychotherapy patients were women, while 60 percent of all new patients in psychotherapy each year were women.

What Feminists Have to Say

Feminist critics of the psychiatric profession observe that the symptoms composing depression in women, for example, are in fact feminine behaviors that were adopted to survive under sexist, oppressive conditions. Real oppression of women causes real distress and unhappiness. Feminist scholars also note the following:

- As late as the 1970s, there was limited social tolerance for women who behaved differently than what was expected within their social roles (and hence, they were judged to be neurotic, psychotic, and so on). That is, women were frequently perceived as "sick" when they rejected the female role (and frequently, when they accepted the role and adopted passive behavior, they were *also* told they were "sick").

- Women in urban North America (which favored the "nuclear" family over the extended family) who outlived their husbands, and who reached menopause, were left "unemployed" at an early age. With the extended family shrinking after World War II, they were left without a family to rear; there was no role for women.

- Women tend to seek help more than men and tend to report their distress more willingly than men.

These three factors helped mobilize women into psychiatrists' offices to seek help for feeling "unfulfilled" with the role of wife and mother. And these feelings can be exacerbated premenstrually.

Not as many women are being sent to mental hospitals as in the past, but many more women are being drugged for their feelings and behaviors. In 2000, Canadian pharmacists issued over 13 million prescriptions for antidepressants — an enormous number when you consider our population size — *and two-thirds of those prescriptions were for women.*

If You Still Want to See a Psychiatrist ...

If you see a psychiatrist for your PMS, you'll be asked to show him or her your PMS chart to see whether your premenstrual discomforts occur seven to ten days prior to your period and then disappear right after, ensuring that you're a perfect candidate for the label "premenstrual dysphoric disorder." So be prepared for a lecture in brain chemistry, depression, and a logical, technical explanation for why you need antidepressants to treat your PMS ... and worse, why you need to take them for the rest of your life! Even if you have been diagnosed with an underlying depression, **there are alternatives to antidepressants**. In the section "How to Say No to Antidepressants" in Chapter 9, "Prescription Drugs used for PMS," where antidepressants are discussed in more detail, I have provided you with a script you can use to help you ask the right questions if this sort of discussion comes up.

Gynecologists and PMS

A gynecologist will also want to look at your PMS charts (see Chapters 3 and 4) to see how your premenstrual discomforts relate to your cycle. Gynecologists will probably recommend hormonal treatments for your PMS before they rule out other conditions or review your diet or lifestyle habits. If you're under 35 and are not planning to get pregnant, expect a prescription for an oral contraceptive, which often does help alleviate the severity of premenstrual discomforts. If you're over 35, don't smoke, and are otherwise healthy, you'll get a prescription for the Pill, too. If you're perimenopausal, you may be given a prescription for either the Pill or hormone replacement therapy. But there are other side effects of oral contraceptives you may not want, and as discussed in the previous chapter, they can wreak havoc on your blood sugar levels.

If hormone therapy is being suggested, be sure to ask whether you can first rule out all of the conditions I discuss in Chapter 4, "The Physical Premenstrual Signs." Try some modifications and adjustments I suggest in Chapters 6 and 7. If you're still suffering, then explore whether your gynecologist is open to natural progesterone therapy, which I discuss in Chapter 8. If your gynecologist wants to put you on an antidepressant, see the section in Chapter 9 called "How to Say No to Antidepressants."

Questionable Gynecological Treatments for PMS

If your gynecologist recommends any of the following treatments for PMS, get another opinion, or better yet, just get *out* of that office.

Hysterectomy.

In general, be wary of any doctor that recommends a hysterectomy for fibroid tumors, as a means for permanent sterilization, to prevent cancer, for cervicitis (inflammation of the cervix), for mildly abnormal patterns of uterine bleeding, for most cases of menstrual pain or PMS, or for abortion during the first and second trimesters.

Ovary Removal.

The only case in which you need your ovaries removed is to prevent the spread of ovarian cancer, or, if there's a damn good reason, to prevent the development of ovarian cancer. Cysts on the ovary, by the way, can be usually be removed, leaving the ovary intact.

D&Cs.

Many years ago, stretching out the uterus via a dilation and curettage (D&C) was considered a treatment for menstrual cramps. Once we discovered painkillers and anti-inflammatories, this practice stopped. A D&C is rarely necessary for most gynecological problems, but is especially *not* appropriate for PMS.

Severing Nerves to Alleviate Pain.

Severing nerves to the uterus and pelvis is a 50-year-old operation popular in some parts of North America. Partially cutting nerves for relieving painful period cramps or endometriosis is a controversial procedure, and there isn't enough research available on this operation to support it.

Menopause-Inducing Hormone Therapy.

Prescribing menopause-inducing hormone therapy, such as Danazol, is just bad medicine and is a sign that your gynecologist is stuck in the 1970s. If this procedure is being recommended for endometriosis, see Chapter 2, "Cycle-Logical Matters."

Endocrinologists and PMS

An endocrinologist will also want to see your charts. The good news, here, is that you're in the right place if you want to rule out blood sugar and thyroid problems first. So do that, along with the all the other "ruling out" conditions described in Chapter 4, "The Physical Premenstrual Signs." Then try to make some of the modifications and changes I suggest in Chapter 6, "The Diet and Exercise Approach," and Chapter 7, "An Herbal and Hands-on Approach." The endocrinologist will probably recommend hormone therapy, and then you can pretty much expect the same treatment approach as a gynecologist's, described above. If this is the case, ask about natural progesterone therapy, which I discuss in Chapter 8. If your endo wants to put you on antidepressants, see the section "How to Say No to Antidepressants" in Chapter 9, "Prescription Drugs Used for PMS."

Primary Care Doctors and PMS

There is a lot of confusion over what constitutes a primary care doctor. So, first, here is a list of some common practitioners who are used for primary care:

- **A general practitioner.** This is an MD with four years of medical school and one year of internship.

- **A family practitioner.** This is an MD with four years of medical school and up to three years of residency training in general or family medicine.

- **An internist.** This is an MD with four years of medical school and up to three years residency training in treatment of illnesses that do not require surgery.

PMS can be managed by a good primary doctor, who, these days, will probably be familiar with diet and lifestyle approaches to PMS. Many family doctors take extra training in naturopathy and alternative medicine, especially when dealing with a large population of female patients. A family practitioner or internist's *job* is to act as your "general contractor," overseeing and project-managing your entire health scenario, looking at "big picture" stuff such as diet, lifestyle, and so on. Their "specialty" is to *generalize* and assess when to call in the "experts." When it's time for a special job, they'll *refer* you to a gynecologist, nutritionist, endocrinologist, oncologist (cancer specialists), physical therapist — whoever. In Canada, primary care doctors can now refer you to homeopaths, naturopaths, and a number of hands-on healers, too, although many of these practitioners are not covered by the provinces' health plans. Primary care doctors can also prescribe natural progesterone therapy, if you've ruled out other conditions and changes to your diet or lifestyle have not reduced your discomfort.

Primary Care Robots versus Doctors

There are quite a few primary care doctors who approach PMS with the standard line they've been fed by antidepressant manufacturers. I call these doctors "robots" who are just trained to memorize diagnostic criteria and refer you to the specialist in that area, or give you a prescription for the latest drug on the market for that condition. That includes antidepressants. All doctors, regardless of specialty or training, can now prescribe antidepressants, even if they haven't been trained at all in psychiatry or psychotherapy. They may quickly refer you to a psychiatrist or just hand out a prescription for an antidepressant. If this is the case, simply say "no thanks" and ask for a referral to a naturopath if possible. Or, see the section in Chapter 9 on how to say no to antidepressants.

Naturopaths, Homeopaths, and PMS

Naturopathy encompasses a broad spectrum of natural therapies. In fact, two colleges in the United States and one in Canada grant the degree of Naturopathic Doctor (ND). Naturopathy is not any one tradition of healing but, instead, it's an umbrella term that refers to an entire array of healing approaches, all based on the body's intrinsic healing powers. This approach tends to appeal to people who distrust prescription medications or are interested in preventative therapies.

NDs will aim to educate their patients about proper lifestyles that can help to avoid degenerative diseases, such as osteoporosis, for example. In many ways, advice from NDs will probably not differ much from the advice of conventional doctors regarding low-fat, high-fiber diets, stress reduction, and so on. However, instead of prescribing an antidepressant, they will more likely aim to treat through nutritional means. They instill the belief that prescription drugs are costly (not just financially), and encourage reliance on natural medicine, including acupuncture, herbs, hydrotherapy, homeopathy, vitamin and mineral supplements, and so on.

To find out about you, all naturopaths and homeopaths will do a thorough history that may last as long as two hours. They'll ask what stresses are going on in your life, what other health problems you have, and so on. They will take the same approach as this book: look at *other* reasons for emotional distress and social causes for depression, *other* causes for general stress and fatigue, *other* conditions that can exacerbate PMS, and so on. They will discuss nutritional and herbal approaches first, along with some lifestyle modifications. If all that fails, they may recommend natural progesterone therapy. You'd be hard-pressed to find an ND or homeopath who recommends antidepressants. You'll find more on homeopathy in Chapter 7, "An Herbal and Hands-on Approach."

Alternative and Complementary Healers

A host of alternative or complementary systems of healing are available to aid in general health and well-being, which can be combined with diet and lifestyle modification or herbal therapies. These systems can also work with other approaches, including hormonal therapy. This section offers you a quick glance into the types of complementary healing available to you, discussed in alphabetical order. (We would need to devote a separate book to really cover this topic, but this will introduce you to the basics!)

Acupuncture

Acupuncture is an ancient Chinese healing art that aims to restore the smooth flow of life energy or *qi* in your body. Acupuncturists believe that your *qi* can be accessed from various points on your body, such as your ear, for example. Each point is also associated with a specific organ. An acupuncturist will use a fine needle on a very specific point, depending on your physical health, to restore *qi* to various organs. Stimulating each of the roughly 2000 points on your body has a specific therapeutic effect. The U.S. National Institute of Health (NIH) is funding research that studies the effects of acupuncture on depression, attention-deficit disorder, hypersensitivity disorder, osteoarthritis, and postoperative dental pain. In one large study, acupuncture offered short-term relief to between 50 and 80 percent of patients with acute or chronic pain. It's now believed that acupuncture stimulates the release of endorphins, which is why it's effective at reducing pain. And that could help alleviate premenstrual aches and pains, too.

Ayurveda

Ayurveda is an ancient Indian approach to health and wellness that has stood up quite well to the test of time. It's roughly 3000 years old. Essentially, it divides up the universe into three basic constitutions or "energies," known as *doshas*. The three doshas are based on wind (*Vata*), fire (*Pitta*), and earth (*Kapha*). These doshas also govern our bodies, personalities, and activities. So while one person is predominantly "Kapha" — thicker in build, often overweight, and more lethargic; another may be predominantly "Vata" — thinner in build, usually with a more finicky appetite and a more hyper personality; or "Pitta" — medium in build with a "hot" constitution and a propensity for spicy foods. When our doshas are balanced all functions well, but when they are not balanced, a state of disease (dis-ease as in "not at ease") can set in. Finding the balance involves changing your diet to suit your predominant dosha (foods are classified as kapha, vata, or pitta, and we eat more or less of whatever we need to achieve balance), doing certain yoga exercises, meditation, and avoiding or incorporating certain lifestyle habits.

An Ayurvedic practitioner will determine your constitution by your appearance, lifestyle habits, and overall personality traits. In addition, the tongue is considered a "map" to the organs and can inform a practitioner what part of the body is unbalanced.

Chinese Medicine

Chinese medicine is roughly 4000 years old. In the same way that Ayurvedic medicine bases the universe on three constitutions, Chinese medicine bases the entire universe on two: yin and yang. Temperaments, organs, foods, activities, and individual personalities are yin or yang. Yang is considered a male constitution, while yin is female. But in all individuals, both yin and yang co-exist. In addition to yin and yang, there are five elements (similar to "doshas" in Ayurvedic medicine) that are based on fire, earth, wood, metal, and water. Different organs in our bodies correspond to different elements. Similar to Ayervedic practice, when everything is balanced, all is healthy and the life force (*qi* – pronounced "chi") flows uninterrupted; when all is not balanced, *qi* can be disturbed and disease can set in. So, finding the balance is the goal of Chinese medicine. To restore balance, diet is either adjusted or supplemented with herbs, pressure points in your body are stimulated through acupuncture (part of Chinese medicine) or massage, and your lifestyle habits may require change as well.

Chiropractic

Chiropractic is gaining acceptance, but your health insurer will consider it an alternative therapy. The word "chiropractic" comes from the Greek *chiro* and *prakrikos*, which means "done by hand." Chiropractic is a tradition that was perfected in the late 1800s by Daniel David Palmer, of Port Perry, Ontario. He was a self-taught healer who eventually founded a practice in Iowa. He believed that all drugs were harmful and his theory was that disease is caused by vertebrae impinging on spinal nerves.

Chiropractors believe that the brain sends energy to every organ along the nerves that run through the spinal cord. When the vertebrae of the spinal column get displaced through stress, poor posture, and so on, this can block or interfere with normal nerve transmission. These interferences are known as "subluxations." In order to cure disease in the body, the chiropractor must remove blockages through adjustments — quick thrusts, massages, and pressures along your spinal column — which move the spinal vertebrae back to normal positions.

Sometimes adjustments involve manipulating the head and extremities (elbows, ankles, knees). This is mostly done by hand, but chiropractors also use special devices to aid them in treatment. A chiropractor will take your medical history, do a general physical exam, and may X-ray your spine to look for misalignments.

Environmental Medicine

Environmental medicine is still considered an "alternative" medicine, even though, in light of what I've revealed in Chapter 4, it probably should be incorporated into conventional practice. Nevertheless environmental medicine is a subspecialty of the allergy and immunology field, which sometimes is called "clinical ecology." An environmental medicine practitioner will look at the impact of environmental factors on your individual health, particularly focusing on the foods, chemicals, water pesticides as well as indoor and outdoor air quality surrounding your life. Treatment usually involves a "clean-up" of whatever is affecting you: diet, air quality (by moving, getting air filters, and so on). Sometimes drugs are prescribed to treat specific allergies, but only in minimal doses.

Iridology

No healer believes that the eyes are "windows to the soul" more than an iridologist, who "reads" the iris. Iridology is not really a therapy but a diagnostic tool used by a wide variety of non-Western healers. Iridology observes changes in texture and color of the iris and correlates them with your physical and mental state of health. An iridologist may tell you not only about an unsuspected thyroid problem, but also that you have an unhealthy relationship with your spouse. Many people have found the experience very accurate and helpful.

Iridology is also used to identify dietary deficiencies and accumulation of toxic chemicals in the body. In fact, in the same way that a Western doctor may send you for a blood test, a natural medicine doctor may send you to an iridologist to expand a diagnosis.

Originally developed by Ignatz von Peczely, a Hungarian physician, in the 19th century, iridology was adapted for modern practice in the 1950s by Bernard Jensen, an American chiropractor. Jensen based his practice on detailed diagrams of the left and right irises. He then assigned every organ, many body parts, and bodily functions to a specific location on one or both irises.

Iridologists believe that the degrees of light and darkness in the iris give enormous clues to the body's general health. They also examine textures of fibers in the iris. Of course, Ayurvedic or Chinese practitioners will also examine the eyes, not just for nearsightedness but for clues to the body's general health. Iridologists will counsel you about nutrition or life habits, but, for the most part, will send you elsewhere for treatment.

Massage Therapy

Massage therapy can be beneficial whether you're receiving massage from your spouse or a massage therapist trained in any one of dozens of techniques from shiatsu to Swedish massage.

All the many forms of massage were developed from shiatsu in the East and Swedish massage in the West. In the East, massage was extensively written about in *The Yellow Emperor's Classic of Internal Medicine,* published in 2700 B.C. (the text that frames the entire Chinese medicine tradition). In Chinese medicine, massage is recommended as a treatment for a variety of illnesses. Swedish massage, the method Westerners are used to experiencing, was developed in the 19th century by a Swedish doctor and poet, Per Henrik, who borrowed techniques from ancient Egypt, China, and Rome. While the philosophies and styles differ in each tradition, the common element is the same: to mobilize the natural healing properties of the body, which will help it maintain or restore optimal health.

Shiatsu-inspired massage focuses on balancing the life force (*qi*). Swedish-inspired massage works on more physiological principles: relaxing muscles to improve blood flow throughout connective tissues, which ultimately strengthens the cardiovascular system.

But no matter what kind of massage you have, numerous gliding and kneading techniques are used, along with deep circular movements and vibrations that relax muscles, improve circulation, and increase mobility. This is known to help relieve stress and often muscle and joint pain. In fact, some employers cover massage therapy in their health plans. See Chapter 7 for more on massage therapy for PMS.

Mind/Body Medicine

Mind/body medicine is a discipline in which physicians, therapists, or other health care providers draw upon traditions of the East to heal their Western clients. They use a variety of techniques, such as meditation, relaxation training, imagery, biofeedback, and breath therapy to help you heal yourself. These techniques are designed for you to "take away" and practice on your own, so that you're not dependent on going to the practitioner every time you need a "fix." An excellent book on mind/body medicine is *Healing Mind, Healthy Woman* by Alice Domar and Henry Dreher.

Reflexology

Reflexology is a 20th century version of an ancient healing and relaxation technique that's probably as old as or older than acupuncture. Western reflexology was developed by Dr. William Fitzgerald, an American ear, nose, and throat specialist, who talked about reflexology as "zone therapy." In fact, reflexology is practiced in several cultures, including Egypt, India, Africa, China, and Japan. In the same way as the ears are a map to the organs, here the feet play the same role, with valuable pressure points that stimulate the life force.

In a nutshell, the "sole is *qi* ('life force') to the soul." By applying pressure to certain parts of the feet, reflexologists can ease pain and tension and restore the body's life force, be it *qi* in China, or *prana* in India.

Reflexologists don't limit themselves to the feet, however. They will also work on hands and ears, although the feet are the most common site. Like most Eastern healing arts, reflexology aims to release the flow of energy through the body along its various pathways. When this energy is trapped for some reason, illness can result. When the energy is released, the body can begin to heal itself.

A reflexologist views the foot as a microcosm of the entire body. Individual reference points or reflex areas on the foot correspond to all major organs, glands, and other parts of the body. Applying pressure to a specific area of the foot stimulates the movement of energy to the corresponding body part. To find a good reflexology map that shows you where to work your own pressure points, visit Dwight D. Byers' website, **www.reflexology-usa.net**. Byers, who uses the famous "Ingham Method" and trains other reflexologists, is considered the foremost reflexology expert.

Are There Risks?

It's important to keep in mind that when it comes to researching alternative therapies, most Western researchers don't know enough about them to design proper studies. And many of these ancient disciplines just don't lend themselves well to Western-style research, such as double-blind, controlled studies. There are other risks with non-Western medicine that you should be aware of:

- There is no scientific proof to support most of the treatments or claims of the therapies you'll be offered.

- Since no advisory board or set of guidelines governs non-Western practitioners, the alternative health care "industry" attracts quacks and charlatans. As well, costs for some therapies may be prohibitive.

- Academic credentials are all over the map in this industry. Beware humbugs.

- Certain preparations are boiled down in clay or metal pots, leaving residues of lead, mercury, arsenic, gold, or cadmium. And it's been reported that sometimes

Chinese herbal preparations are laced with prescription drugs. Be careful and purchase from reputable sources.

- Dosages are all over the map. For example, the active ingredient in many herbs may not be accurately measured. One reason modern medicine moved away from herbal preparations is that manufactured drugs were easier to purify and standardize. When you buy 10 100-mg tablets of any prescription drug, that's what you get. But when you buy 10 capsules of an herb, the dosages may vary from capsule to capsule.

Women Healing Women

When it comes to premenstrual discomforts, other women, who may or not be health care practitioners, are often great sources of information. In fact, women have been healing each other, assisting each other in childbirth (through midwifery), and sharing ingenious reproductive health remedies and recipes since the beginning of time. It's called "girl talk" in lay terms, but fancier terms refer to women healing through "oral tradition" or "narratives." Women can connect on a number of health issues on the Internet through online chat rooms and health forums. The most renowned women's health book and "bible," *Our Bodies, Ourselves,* by the Boston Women's Health Book Collective, is a standard in women's health information that was not created by doctors at all — male or female. It was created through girl talk!

The Boston Women's Health Collective grew out of a course by and for women about health, sexuality, and child-bearing. This small group of women met regularly to discuss aspects of women's health, particularly their frustrations with doctors. When they realized that "the personal was political" in that their experiences mirrored the state of women's health at that time, each woman in the group took a topic, such as abortion or rape, made that the focus of her research, and then brought back what she had learned to the larger group.

Although *Our Bodies, Ourselves* has been revised several times over the last 30 years and has sold over four million copies, it still reflects women's own self-knowledge about their health and is just as relevant today as its first edition in 1970. Says Gloria Steinem:

> I was part of that small demographic slice of people most likely to get the best health care information. As a journalist, I was even in a position to research what I didn't know. Yet what "best" meant in those largely prefeminist days was whatever limited information the medical establishment considered appropriate — for patients in general and for women in particular. (Steinem, Preface to the 25th Anniversary Edition, *Our Bodies, Ourselves: For the New Century, 17.*)

Our Bodies, Ourselves was one of the strongest markers of the Women's Health Movement in North America.

Well Woman Clinics

When women realized that men ought not to be controlling health care for women's bodies, the grassroots women's health movement started health care reform in the 1970s. No longer acceptable were the lack of health information provided, abuse of medical procedures, lack of good birth control information, or being told that natural female processes were diseases. Women were tired of not being in control of their bodies.

"Well woman" clinics run by ordinary women were springing up all over North America in the mid-to-late 1970s. For example, knowledge gained about our own bodies by simply looking at the cervix at different stages proved that much of what women were told about their health status "down there" was false. For example, one women's clinic discovered that although gynecologists told women who had a tipped or retroverted uterus that they were abnormal, it is in fact the most common shape of uterus. Several community-based self-help programs also changed the delivery of women's health care.

The women's health collective model has also been used to change the way psychosocial services are delivered to women. For example, Toronto's Women's Counselling, Referral and Education Centre evolved from concerns amongst feminists and mental health professionals about the over-prescribing of psychotropic drugs to women. This is how feminist therapy came into being (see Chapter 3, "The Emotional Premenstrual Signs," for more on feminist therapy).

Women Watchdogs

The grassroots activism that led to women-created clinics and education over women's health evolved into political action organizations. One such group, California's Coalition for the Medical Rights of Women, started in 1974, has been effective in achieving the regulation and labeling of drugs and medical devices, particularly to protect pregnant women and women's reproductive health.

Professional Women Healers: Witches, Doctors, and Nurses

Women have a long history as activists within the health care profession. As early as the third century B.C., conflicts over female physicians/midwives performing abortions led to public demonstrations by women over the right to practice. In Greece, one protest over a female disguised as a male gynecologist was recorded. The witch-hunts of the 15th and 16th centuries involved branding female healers "witches," while the displacement of female lay healers and midwives throughout the 19th century echoed the ancient conflict over gender rights within the health care system, or rather, who would control health care.

Nursing is a profession that values caring and nurturing, compared to the values of patriarchal and paternalistic medicine, which values curing and scientific research. Nurses can perform many of the same tasks — with greater skill and care — than many male doctors. Although nurses have struggled over issues of credentials, professionalization, and conditions and scope of nursing work, there has not been enough criticism of the structures that support the continued devaluing of nurses

Women medical students in Manitoba reported the following biases and abuses:

- Male-dominated admissions committees

- Admission interview questions to women about their plans for a family, but not to men

- Discouraging comments from professors and clinicians when women expressed interest in pursuing more challenging specialties

- Low percentages of female teachers in medical school (between 5 and 20 percent)

- Language that is more suited to male socialization than female

- Gender-biased student services information

- Devaluing the female body by making the 35-year-old, 70-kilogram male body the norm

- Devaluing women's health issues in lectures

- Nonclinical language used to describe women's bodies and women's health issues by professors while clinical language used to describe the male body (for example, "tits" versus "penis")

- Inappropriate jokes exploiting women told in class by lecturing professors

- Character attacks on women with certain diseases made by professors (for example, "women with PID are promiscuous")

Feminist doctors who graduated medical school and remained in the traditional female doctor specialties of family practice or obstetrics and gynecology have influenced health care practices by consciously applying feminist principles in their practices. That said, just because a doctor is female does not mean she is practicing woman-centered medicine. As well, there are different definitions of woman-centered medicine.

When given a choice, most women prefer to discuss their health problems with another woman. Here are some ways to find women to heal you:

- Join a PMS chat room or forum to compare remedies and see what other women have found helpful.
- Organize a PMS group with co-workers and friends to openly discuss discomforts, remedies, lifestyle issues, and so on. Connecting with other women is also a great way to relieve stress and depression.
- Find a women's community center in your area; these centers usually offer a range of health services, such as counseling and well-woman check-ups (Pap tests, PMS counseling, birth control), and are often supervised by nurses.

What Are Your Rights as a Patient?

Patients' rights in Western health care involve four basic umbrella principles: respect for persons (or patient autonomy), beneficence, nonmaleficence, and justice. Since so many women looking for ways to ease their premenstrual discomforts are put on questionable therapies or dismissed by doctors, this is important information for you to have. You can challenge your doctor on any of these principles, and you can use the following information to launch a complaint to the Royal College of Physicians and Surgeons in your province if you feel your rights have been ignored. This section has been reviewed by experts at the University of Toronto's Joint Centre for Bioethics. For more information, you can also visit my Bioethics Page and links at **www.sarahealth.com**.

Respect for Persons (also Known as Patient Autonomy)

This principle means that the health care provider should respect that each person is, in fact, a human being with full human rights. That means you have a right to be fully informed about all things involving your care, your body, or things being done to your body (if you're pregnant, you also have the right to know about everything that affects the fetus you're carrying), and to make your own decisions about care based on accurate information.

A health care provider has a duty to respect your personhood, wishes, bodily integrity, and health care preferences. Information, counseling, and informed consent (see further on) are all crucial aspects of care that support this principle. Here are some examples of when your health care provider is ignoring respect for persons:

- You are given no information about your condition, and your doctor refuses to answer or address your questions.
- You refuse a certain treatment or procedure after being fully informed of all of the risks and benefits of that procedure, but your health care provider tries to force or coerce you into having the procedure anyway, which does not respect your choice.
- You request a referral to a specialist and your doctor ignores your request.
- You do not speak English and your doctor refuses to speak to a translator you've appointed.
- Your doctor forces a feeding tube up the nose of your 92-year-old mother who suffers from severe dementia, over your express objections as her appointed decision-maker.
- Your confidentiality is breached in some way.

What Is "Informed Consent"?

Many of you have heard the term "informed consent," but you may not truly understand what it means. To uphold the principle of respect for persons, you have the right to accurate and full information about your health so you can make an informed decision about your health care. You cannot even know to refuse a procedure if you are not given this information first. When you are given enough information to make a decision, this is known as informed consent.

Barriers to informed consent include language barriers, wide gaps in knowledge (when you're not a doctor, how informed can you really be unless you go to medical school?), and health care provider bias (when your health care provider makes assumptions about your intelligence or character and tailors the information to those assumptions).

In order for informed consent to take place, three things have to happen: you must have full disclosure of information, you must be capable of understanding and deciding about the information, and you must make your decisions voluntarily.

Disclosure.

Have you been provided with relevant and comprehensive information by your health care provider? Information should include, for example, a description of the treatment; its expected effects (such as duration of hospital stay, expected time to recovery, restrictions on daily activities, scars); information about relevant alternative options and their expected benefits and relevant risks; and an explanation of the consequences of declining or delaying treatment. Have you been given an opportunity to ask questions, and has your health care provider been available to answer them?

Capacity and Competency.
Do you understand information relevant to a treatment decision and appreciate the reasonably foreseeable consequences of a decision or lack of decision? Do you understand information and appreciate its implications? Do you understand what's being disclosed and can you decide on your treatment based on this information?

Voluntariness.
Are you being allowed to make your health care choice free of any undue influences? To answer the question, we need to take into consideration factors such as pain and manipulation (when information is being deliberately distorted or omitted.

What about Confidentiality?

No matter how confidential you think your health care records or the information you disclose to your health care provider are, your medical records are, in fact, not confidential. These are the questions you must ask your health care provider if you're concerned about confidential information getting into the wrong hands:

Who Owns This Information?
For example, if you test positive for a particular cancer gene or HIV, does your health care provider have a duty to report this information to anyone other than yourself? If you're placed on antidepressants, do you want this information to get out? Can you bar your physician from disclosing this information? And what about employers who demand that you have routine physicals?

How Will This Information Be Used?
Can your health status information be used by employers or health insurers as tools of discrimination? In the 1970s, for example, African Americans who were tested positive for sickle cell anemia were denied jobs by major airlines and were forced to pay higher insurance costs.

How Will Your Health Status Affect Other Family Members?
If you test positive for a particular cancer gene, for example, do you have to disclose this information to your children? Ought you? Ought they to be tested? And what are the consequences involved?

Beneficence and Nonmaleficence
(Doing Some Good and Doing No Harm)

Beneficence (pronounced "be-NI-fi-cents") means that the health care provider must strive to maintain or promote the well-being of a patient, and avoid harming that patient. At the same time, the health care provider must also strive not to inflict harm or evil on a patient; this is known as "nonmaleficence" (pronounced "non-mal-IF-i-cents"). This means that a health care provider has a duty not to kill a patient and a duty not to refrain from aiding a patient.

In order to promote the well-being of patients and avoid harming them, therapies, treatments, or diagnostic tests that involve risks to your health need to be weighed against potential benefits. Here are some examples of when your health care provider is ignoring beneficence and nonmaleficence:

- Your doctor recommends you try an experimental therapy that has not yet been proven to work better than a standard therapy, and has unknown risks.
- You are given a drug or therapy and not provided with information on side-effects or potential risks.
- You are in a drug study that involves some people taking a "dummy pill" (called a placebo) and some people taking a real pill. In this case, you may continue to suffer from an ailment needlessly if you are taking the dummy pill and not offered a standard therapy that will help your ailment.
- Your health care provider breaches your confidentiality.

Justice

The principle of justice in providing health care means that the health care provider or system has to ensure that everyone has the same access to health care services (such as hospital beds, medicine, treatments, clinical trials, health care providers, preventive care, and so on) regardless of their ability to pay, gender, ethnicity or race, physical or mental ability, age, or any other factors, such as behavior or lifestyle.

In order to be fair, all people should have equal access to health care services and resources. Being just or fair means all lives and interests are of equal importance and must be given equal weight. As well, a health care provider has a duty to provide the same standard of care and options to all patients, regardless of income, education, or race. Here are some examples of when the health care system — or your individual health care provider — is ignoring justice:

- When some people have more access to resources than other people due to privilege and wealth

- When your health care provider places a greater value on some patients than on others

- When poor women have babies with lower birth weights and more complications at birth than affluent women because they have less access to good prenatal care

- When an HIV-positive person is refused health care service by a health care provider who fears HIV

- When certain groups of people die of curable diseases because they don't have the same access to screening for that disease that other groups of people do

- When vulnerable populations (the elderly, mentally ill, people in developing countries, or certain ethnic groups) are selected for dangerous or risky medical experiments because they are perceived as "expendable"

Problems with "Doing the Right Thing" for Patients

Ignoring one of the above principles can put you in jeopardy, which would make the health care provider negligent. But in many circumstances it isn't always clear what "the right thing" to do is, and it isn't always possible to do the right thing, as these examples illustrate.

- When people are unconscious, for example, it's impossible to inform them and ask them about their wishes. (In this case, someone close to the unconscious person may make decisions on his or her behalf.)

- When people are not competent to make their own decisions, it's difficult to inform them. (Here, again, someone close to the incompetent patient makes the decision.)

- When the benefits of certain medications or therapies have to be weighed against certain risks, it's difficult to know what to do, and what's in the patient's best interests.

- When health care providers are faced with limited resources, such as funding for research, organs for transplant, or even hospital beds, it's difficult to decide who should get the funds, organs, or beds.

- When conducting drug studies, is it right to conduct a study in which someone is taking a dummy pill (known as a placebo-controlled study)?

Whose life is worth saving? Whose life is worth risking? And who decides? These are all common, everyday questions and situations that health care providers face.

Legal Duties of Health Care Providers

Whether health care practitioners are considered to be trained in a conventional or unconventional manner, charging a fee for services ought to imply that there are standards of competence their patients or clients have a right to expect. Any health care professional who earns a salary is bound by tort law to uphold standards of care. Moreover, all health care practitioners have a duty to maintain "due awareness," meaning that they have a duty to stay educated, informed, and up to date on all aspects of legally enforceable duties of care to patients, their families, colleagues, and staff members. Health care providers have a basic duty to diagnose, treat, manage, or care for a health problem. They also have a duty to counsel you about potential harms you may be doing to yourself through medications you're taking, bad habits or other practices, or harms from outside forces beyond your control, such as environmental factors. And finally, when medical records need to be transferred or copied to a third party, health care providers have a duty to disclose potentially sensitive or stigmatizing information to that party, as well as to you.

Health care standards of practice in Canada have two legal checks: you can sue or you can complain to the professional regulatory authority, such as the College of Physicians and Surgeons, which monitors standards of practice to protect the public.

6

THE DIET AND EXERCISE APPROACH

In looking at the physical signs of PMS in Chapter 4, we saw that there are two key things that can be completely solved through diet. The first is that when you're pumping out adrenaline as a result of stress, it prevents progesterone receptors from functioning, which worsens your PMS. Second, low blood sugar blocks progesterone receptors, so by eating steadily throughout the day and keeping your blood sugar levels stable, you can improve PMS. (You also pump out adrenaline when your blood sugar is low.) This, in turn, may improve thyroid function, as progesterone levels are naturally restored.

Mood swings associated with PMS can also be completely solved through diet, as mood swings are exacerbated by low blood sugar. Our brains also require several nutrients to function properly. And finally, exercise creates endorphins, which function as an antidepressant. Eliminating extra stimulants and depressants, such as caffeine and alcohol, prior to your period can also improve PMS. So ... the diet and exercise approach is often the only approach you need to solve your PMS problems.

Stabilizing Your Blood Sugar

The most important step in improving PMS is stabilizing your blood sugar level. Dr. Katharina Dalton recommends the "Three Hourly Starch Diet," which basically means eat something starchy (rice, potatoes, pasta, etc.) every three hours. This is not the only way to stabilize blood sugar levels. Ensuring that you get enough protein, fiber, and fat in your meals will also help to maintain blood sugar levels and delay glucose absorption, which has the same effect.

The kinds of foods you should use as building blocks for your meals are grains and beans; lean meat, fish, and chicken; and fresh fruits and vegetables.

Understanding Carbs Once and For All!

The word *carbohydrates* means "starchy stuff," such as rice, pasta, breads, or potatoes. Carbohydrates can be simple or complex. Simple carbohydrates are found in any food that has natural sugar (honey, fruits, juices, vegetables, milk) and anything that contains table sugar. Complex carbohydrates are more sophisticated foods that are made up of larger molecules, such as grain foods, starches, and foods high in fiber.

Normally, all carbs convert into glucose when you eat them. Glucose is the technical term for "simplest sugar." All your energy comes from glucose in your blood, also known as blood glucose or blood sugar — your body fuel. When your blood sugar is used up, you feel weak and tired ... and hungry. But what happens when you eat more carbohydrates than your body can use? Your body will store those extra carbs as fat.

What we also know is that the rate at which glucose from carbohydrates is absorbed by your body is affected by other parts of your meal, such as the protein, fiber, and fat. If you're eating only carbohydrates and no protein or fat, for example, the carbs will convert into glucose more quickly — to the point where you may feel mood swings as your blood sugar rises and dips.

Nutrition experts today advise that for a healthy diet you should consume roughly 40 percent carbohydrates, 30 percent protein, and 30 percent fat daily. (This was revised even from two years ago, when it was thought that 55 percent of the diet should be composed of carbohydrates.) Some carbohydrates convert into glucose faster than others. Table 6.1 can help you select slower-converting carbohydrates to balance your diet.

TABLE 6.1   How Your Food Breaks Down

Complex Carbohydrates (digests more slowly)

Fruits	Grains (breads, pastas, and cereals)
Vegetables (corn, potatoes, etc.)	Legumes (dried beans, peas, and lentils)

Simple Carbohydrates (digests quickly)

Fruits/fruit juices	Sorghum
Sugars (sucrose, fructose, etc.)	Date sugar
Honey	Molasses
Corn syrup	Lactose

Proteins (digest slowly)

Lean meats	Low-fat cheese
Fatty meats	High-fat cheese
Poultry	Legumes
Fish	Grains
Eggs	

Fats (digest slowly)

High-fat dairy products (butter or cream)	Avocados
Oils (canola/corn/olive/safflower/sunflower)	Olives
Lard	Nuts

Fiber (soluble fiber slows digestion; insoluble fiber helps to form bulk in the stool for easy elimination)

Whole-grain breads	Legumes (beans and lentils)
Cereals (e.g., oatmeal)	Leafy greens
All fruits	Cruciferous vegetables (e.g., broccoli, brussels sprouts, or cauliflower)

A good way to gauge how quickly your food converts to glucose is to use the glycemic index (see Table 6.2). The glycemic index (GI) shows the rise in blood sugar from various carbohydrates. Therefore, planning your diet using the GI can help you control your blood sugar by using more foods with a low GI and fewer foods with a high GI. Nutritionists report that it is useful as a tool in meal planning.

TABLE 6.2   The Glycemic Index at a Glance

This glycemic index, developed at the University of Toronto, measures the rate at which various foods convert to glucose. Higher numbers indicate a more rapid absorption of glucose, which itself is assigned a value of 100. This is not an exhaustive list and should be used as a sample only. This is not an index of food energy values or calories; some low-GI foods are high in fat, while some high-GI foods are low in fat. Keep in mind, too, that these values differ depending upon what else you're eating with that food and how the food is prepared.

Sugars

Glucose = 100	Table sugar = 59
Honey = 87	Fructose = 20

Snacks

Mars Bar = 68	Tomato soup = 38
Potato chips = 51	Sausages = 28
Sponge cake = 46	Peanuts = 13
Fish sticks = 38	

Cereals

Cornflakes = 80	All Bran = 51
Shredded wheat = 67	Oatmeal = 49
Muesli = 66	

Breads

Whole wheat = 72	Buckwheat = 51
White = 69	

Fruits

Raisins = 64	Orange = 40
Banana = 62	Apple = 39
Orange juice = 46	

Dairy Products

Ice cream = 36	Milk (regular fat) = 34
Yogurt = 36	Skim milk = 32

TABLE 6.2 <u>The Glycemic Index at a Glance</u> (continued)

Root Vegetables

Parsnips = 97	Beets = 64
Carrots = 92	Yam = 51
Instant mashed potatoes = 80	Sweet potato = 48
New boiled potato = 70	

Pasta and Rice

White rice = 72	Spaghetti (white) = 50
Brown rice = 66	Spaghetti (whole wheat) = 42

Legumes

Frozen peas = 51	Black-eyed peas = 33
Baked beans = 40	Green beans = 31
Chickpeas = 36	Kidney beans = 29
Lima beans = 36	Lentils = 29
Butter beans = 36	Dried soybeans = 15

Carbs and Low-Fat Diets

Low-fat diets may also contribute to PMS because they promote insulin resistance. In a low-fat diet, most of your calories come from carbohydrates rather than protein or fat. Carbohydrates convert into glucose quickly in the body. So you eat, feel full, and then feel very hungry again. In order to feel satisfied and satiated, we must have some fat in our diets. But in addition, fat in our diets also trigger fat-burning compounds in our bodies. Years of conditioning us to "no fat" has made most people fatter and has dramatically increased our risk of developing blood sugar problems because of the amount of insulin we require to "clean up" the carbohydrates that convert so quickly into sugar.

A whole industry of diet books promotes low-carbohydrate or no-carbohydrate diets, such as *Dr. Atkins' New Diet Revolution*, *Protein Power* and *The Zone*. But many nutrition experts consider the diets promoted in these books to be dangerous. The Dr. Atkins diet is dangerous because it is based on a huge amount of saturated fat, which is the major source of "bad cholesterol" in the diet. Regardless of how much weight you may lose on the Atkins diet, you are still at risk for heart disease because of the saturated fat and high LDL (low-density lipids) levels. The Zone diet, according to some experts, has no scientific basis. The book claims that high carbs and insulin make you fat when, in fact, it is calories from all sources of food that make you fat when you don't output the energy needed to burn them off.

Carbohydrates and Moods

One of the most important factors in diet and moods is your blood sugar level. Many women, for example, find they suffer from repeated episodes of low blood sugar, known as *hypoglycemia*. This is usually caused by consuming too many carbohydrates, which produces an initial "rush" of energy followed by a tremendous "crash," which is sometimes known as postprandial depression (or postmeal depression). In fact, during episodes of depression, it's not at all unusual to crave simple carbohydrates, such as sugars and sweets. The simpler the carbohydrate, the faster it breaks down into glucose and the faster the drop in blood sugar, leading to a drop in mood. People with seasonal affective disorder (see Chapter 3) are especially known to crave sugars, such as chocolate and candy. The cravings for sweets are so powerful in SAD (80 percent of those with SAD have these cravings), that many doctors consider it a symptom of SAD.

If you think you suffer from low blood sugar, schedule an appointment with a nutritionist through your primary care physician and plan a diet that is based on a variety of foods rather than mostly carbohydrates. By increasing your intake of protein and fiber, you can help to delay the breakdown of your food into glucose, which will keep your blood sugar levels more stable throughout the day.

Reading Food Labels

Understanding what you're buying can be challenging when you're carb-counting. The aisles of a supermarket are not only the aisles of temptation, they may have foods with complicated food labels. In Canada, ingredients on labels are listed according to weight, with the "most" listed first. If sugar is the first ingredient, you know the product contains mostly sugar. The lower sugar is on the list, the less sugar in the product. The nutrition information on the label should also list the total amount of carbohydrates in a *serving* of the food. That amount includes both natural and added sugars.

When a label says the product is "calorie-reduced" or "carbohydrate-reduced," that means there are 50 percent less calories or carbohydrates compared to the original product. But something that was originally 7,000 calories isn't much better at 3,500!

"Cholesterol-free" or "low cholesterol" means that the product doesn't have any, or much, animal fat (hence, cholesterol). This doesn't mean "low fat." Pure vegetable oil doesn't come from animals but it is pure fat!

A label that screams "low fat" means that the product has less than 3 grams of fat per serving. In potato-chip country, that means about six potato chips. *(I don't know anybody who ate only one serving of potato chips!)* So if you eat the whole bag of "low-fat" chips, you're still eating a lot of fat. Be sure to check serving sizes.

Products that are "light" (or "lite") mean that there is 25 to 50 percent less of some ingredient in that product. It could be fat, cholesterol, salt, or sugar, or less food coloring, and therefore the designation is frequently misleading.

"Sugar-Free."

Careful! Sugar-free in the language of labels simply means "sucrose-free." That does not mean the product is *carbohydrate free*, as in dextrose-free, lactose-free, glucose-free, or fructose-free. Check the labels for all things ending in "ose" to find out the sugar content; you're not just looking for sucrose. Watch out for "no added sugar," "without added sugar," or "no sugar added." This simply means: "We didn't put the sugar in, God did." Again, reading the amount of carbohydrates on the nutrition information label is the most accurate way to know the amount of sugar in the product. Nutrition claims in big, bold statements can be misleading.

"Less and More."

Then there are the comparison claims, such as "fewer," "reduced," "less," "more," or, my favorite — "light" (or worse, "lite"!). These words appear on foods that have been nutritionally altered from a previous "version" or competitor's version. For example, *Brand X Potato Chips — Regular* may have much more fat than *Brand X Potato Chips — Lite*, "with less fat than Regular Brand X." That doesn't mean that Brand X Lite is fat-free, or even low in fat. It just means it's *lower* in fat than Brand X Regular.

On the flip side, *Brand Y* may have a trace amount of calcium, while *Brand Y+*, *"now with more calcium"* may still have a small amount of calcium, but 10 percent more than Brand Y. (In other words, you may still need to eat 100 bowls of Brand Y+ before you get the daily requirement for calcium!)

To be light or "lite" in fat, a product has to contain either one-third fewer calories or half the fat of the regular product. Something that is "light in sodium" means it has at least 50 percent less sodium than the regular product, such as canned soup. (But if you're buying hair coloring that reads "light brown," it is a descriptive word, not referring to an ingredient!)

Born in the U.S.A.

American labels that say "sugar-free" mean the product contains less than 0.5 grams of sugar per serving, while a "reduced-sugar" food contains at least 25 percent less sugar per serving than the regular product. If the label also states that the product is not a reduced- or low-calorie food, or it is not for weight control, it's got enough sugar in there to make you think twice.

Serving sizes in the United States are also listed differently. Foods that are similar are given the same *type* of serving size defined by the U.S. Food and Drug Administration (FDA). This means that five cereals that each weigh 10 grams per cup will share the same serving sizes.

Calories (the amount of energy) and calories from fat (the amount of fat) are also listed per serving of food in the United States. Total carbohydrate, dietary fiber, sugars, other carbohydrates (which means starches), total fat, saturated fat, cholesterol, sodium, potassium, and vitamin and minerals are given in percentages based on the Recommended Daily Allowance values, based on the 2,000-calorie diet recommended by the U.S. government. In Canada, Recommended Nutrient Intake (RNI) is used for vitamins and minerals.

Fake Fat.

We have artificial sweeteners; why not artificial fat? This question has led to the creation of an emerging yet highly suspicious ingredient: *fat substitute*, designed to replace real fat and hence reduce the calories from real fat without compromising the taste. This is done by creating a fake fat that the body cannot absorb.

One of the first fat substitutes was Simplesse, made from milk and egg-white protein, which was developed by the NutraSweet Company. Simplesse apparently adds 1 to 2 calories per gram instead of the usual 9 calories per gram from fat. Other fat substitutes simply take protein and carbohydrates and modify them in some way to simulate the textures of fat (creamy, smooth, etc.) All of these fat substitutes help to create low-fat products.

Procter & Gamble is now promoting a new calorie-free fat substitute they developed called olestra. It's currently being test marketed in the United States in a variety of savory snacks such as potato chips and crackers. Olestra is a potentially dangerous ingredient that most experts feel can do more harm than good. Canada has not yet approved it.

Olestra is made from a combination of vegetable oils and sugar. Therefore, it tastes just like the real thing, but the biochemical structure is a molecule too big for your liver to break down. So, olestra just passes into the large intestine and is excreted. Olestra is more than an "empty" molecule, however. According to the FDA Commissioner of Food and Drugs, olestra may cause diarrhea and cramps and may deplete your body of vital nutrients, including vitamins A, D, E, and K (necessary for blood to clot). And indeed, all studies conducted by Procter & Gamble have shown this potential.

If the FDA approves olestra for use as a cooking-oil substitute, you'll see it in every imaginable high-fat product. But nutritionists pointed out another danger with olestra in a critique published in *The University of California at Berkeley Wellness Letter* in 1996 (the year olestra was approved for test markets). Instead of encouraging people to choose nutritious foods, such as fruits, grains, and vegetables, over high-fat foods, products like olestra encourage a high *fake*-fat diet that's still too low in fiber and other essential nutrients. And the no-fat icing on the cake is that these people could potentially wind up with a vitamin deficiency, to boot. Products like olestra should make you nervous.

Sweeteners

Here's what you need to know about sweeteners if you're trying to cut down on fat. While artificial sweeteners do not contain sugar (for diabetics, this means they will not affect blood sugar levels), they *may* contain a tiny amount of calories. It depends upon whether that sweetener is classified as nutritive or non-nutritive.

Nutritive sweeteners have calories or contain natural sugar. White or brown table sugar, molasses, honey, and syrup are all considered nutritive sweeteners. *Sugar alcohols* are also nutritive sweeteners because they are made from fruits or produced commercially from dextrose (which is just edible glucose). Sorbitol, mannitol, xylitol, and maltitol are all sugar alcohols. Sugar alcohols contain only 4 calories per gram, like ordinary sugar, and will affect your blood sugar levels in the same way as ordinary sugar. It all depends on how much is consumed, and the degree of absorption from your digestive tract.

Non-nutritive sweeteners are sugar substitutes or artificial sweeteners; they do not have any calories and will not affect your blood sugar levels. Examples of non-nutritive sweeteners are saccharin, cyclamate, aspartame, sucralose, and acesulfame potassium.

The Sweetener Wars

The oldest non-nutritive sweetener is saccharin, which is what you get when you purchase Sweet'N Low or Hermesetas. In Canada, saccharin can be used only as a table-top sweetener in either tablet or powder form. Saccharin is 300 times sweeter than sucrose (table sugar) but has a metallic aftertaste. In the 1970s, saccharin was also thought to cause cancer, but this was never proven.

In the 1980s, aspartame was invented, which is sold as NutraSweet. It was considered a nutritive sweetener because it was derived from natural sources (two amino acids, aspartic acid and phenylalanine), which means that aspartame is digested and metabolized the same way as any other protein foods. For every gram of aspartame, there are 4 calories. But since aspartame is 200 times sweeter than sugar, you don't need very much of it to achieve the desired sweetness. In at least 90 countries, aspartame is found in more than 150 product categories, including breakfast cereals, beverages, desserts, candy and gum, syrups, salad dressings, and various snack foods. Here's where it gets confusing: aspartame is also available as a tabletop sweetener under the brand name Equal, and most recently, PROSWEET. An interesting point about aspartame is that it's not recommended for baking or any other recipe that requires heat. The two amino acids in it separate with heat and the product loses its sweetness. That's not to say it's harmful if heated, but your recipe won't turn out.

For the moment, aspartame is considered safe for everybody, including people with diabetes, pregnant women, and children. The only people who are cautioned against consuming it are those with a rare hereditary disease known as phenylketonuria (PKU) because aspartame contains phenylalanine, which people with PKU cannot tolerate.

Another common tabletop sweetener is sucralose, sold as Splenda. Splenda is a white crystalline powder, actually made from sugar itself. It's 600 times sweeter than table sugar but is not broken down in your digestive system, so it has no calories at all. Splenda can be used in hot or cold foods and is found in hot and cold beverages, frozen foods, baked goods, and other packaged foods.

Cyclamate, a non-nutritive sweetener, is the sweetener used in many weight control products and is 30 times sweeter than table sugar, with no aftertaste. Cyclamate is fine for hot or cold foods. In the United States, you can purchase cyclamate under the brand name Sucaryl or Sugar Twin. In Canada, however, you can only find cyclamate as Sugar Twin or as a sugar substitute in medication.

The Newest Sweeteners

The newest addition to the sweetener industry is acesulfame potassium (Ace-K), recently approved by Health Canada. About 200 times sweeter than table sugar, Ace-K is sold as Sunett and is found in beverages, fruit spreads, baked goods, dessert mixes, tabletop sweeteners, hard candies, chewing gum, and breath fresheners. While no specific studies on Ace-K and diabetes have been done, the only people who are cautioned against ingesting Ace-K are those on a potassium-restricted diet or people who are allergic to sulpha drugs.

Researchers at the University of Maryland have discovered another sweetener that can be specifically designed for people with diabetes. This sweetener would be based on D-tagatose, a hexose sugar found naturally in yogurt, cheese, or sterilized milk. The beauty of this ingredient is that D-tagatose has no effect on insulin levels or blood sugar levels in people with and without diabetes. Experts believe that D-tagatose delays the absorption of carbohydrates.

D-tagatose looks identical to fructose, and has about 92 percent of the sweetness of sucrose, except only 25 percent of it will be metabolized. Currently, D-tagatose is being developed as a bulk sweetener. It is a few years away from being marketed and sold as a brand-name sweetener, however.

Sugar Alcohols

Not to be confused with alcoholic beverages, sugar alcohols are nutritive sweeteners, like regular sugar. These are found naturally in fruits or manufactured from carbohydrates. Sorbitol, mannitol, xylitol, maltitol, maltitol syrup, lactitol, isomalt, and hydrogenated starch hydrolysates are all sugar alcohols. In your body, these types of sugars are absorbed lower down in the digestive tract and will cause gastrointestinal symptoms if you use too much. Because sugar alcohols are absorbed more slowly, they were once touted as ideal for people with diabetes, but, since they are a carbohydrate, they still increase your blood sugar — just like regular sugar. Now that artificial sweeteners are on the market in abundance, the only real advantage of sugar alcohols is that they don't cause cavities. The bacteria in your mouth doesn't like sugar alcohols as much as real sugar.

According to the FDA, even foods that contain sugar alcohols can be labeled "sugar-free." Sugar alcohol products can also be labeled "Does not promote tooth decay," which is often confused with "low-calorie."

Diet, Stress, and Depression

We now know there are a variety of daily nutrients that help to regulate our stress levels and moods. Tryptophan, for example, which is found in milk and other dairy products, helps our bodies to build neurotransmitters, such as serotonin. Tryptophan is sometimes used separately as an "augmenter" to boost the effect of antidepressant medication.

The B vitamins are also important for our mental health. Vitamin B_{12} is crucial for good general health, while other B-complex vitamins (thiamine, riboflavin, niacin, pyridoxine, pantothenic acid, and biotin) are essential for brain function, enabling you to be cognizant and alert. You'll find the B vitamins in lean meats, whole grains, liver, seeds, nuts, wheat germ, and dairy products. Folate (a.k.a. folic acid) is particularly important for a healthy mood. It is found in liver, eggs, leafy greens, yeast, legumes, whole grains, nuts, fruits (bananas, orange juice, grapefruit juice), and vegetables (broccoli, spinach, asparagus, brussels sprouts). When you don't have enough "brain foods" you can become more prone to depression.

Calcium and magnesium are also linked to mood — and, not surprisingly, PMS. Both of these nutrients aid in the proper transmission of nerve impulses. Calcium is found in dairy products, leafy greens, eggs, and fish (particularly salmon and sardines). Soy, nuts, whole grains, milk, meat, and fish contain magnesium. Calcium, the biggest news in PMS supplements, is discussed further on.

Foods to Avoid during PMS

Removing PMS irritants such as sugar, salt, caffeine, and alcohol about two weeks before your period is a good way to reduce the severity of premenstrual changes. As I discuss in Chapter 4, "The Physical Premenstrual Signs," sugar can increase your blood sugar and cause sugar highs and crashes; caffeine is a stimulant that can increase your irritability and stress levels; while alcohol is a depressant that may contribute to an already depressed mood during PMS. Salt causes you to retain water, so reducing your salt intake will help reduce bloating. Drinking more water will also help to eliminate bloat.

What You Should Know about Sugar

Sugar is one of the hardest things to reduce since it's in a lot of foods we don't expect. Sugars are found naturally in many foods you eat. The simplest form of sugar is glucose, which is what "blood sugar" (also called "blood glucose") is — your basic body fuel. You can buy pure glucose at any drugstore in the form of dextrose tablets. Dextrose is just "edible glucose." For example, when people are fed "sugar water" intravenously, dextrose is the sugar in that water. When you see "dextrose" on a candy-bar label, it means that the candy-bar manufacturer used "edible glucose" in the recipe.

Glucose is the baseline ingredient of all naturally occurring sugars, which include the following:

- **Sucrose:** table or white sugar, naturally found in sugar cane and sugar beets
- **Fructose:** the natural sugar in fruits and vegetables
- **Lactose:** the natural sugar in all milk products
- **Maltose:** the natural sugar in grains (flours and cereals)

When you ingest a natural sugar of any kind, you're actually ingesting one part glucose and one or two parts of *another* naturally occurring sugar. For example, sucrose is biochemically constructed from one part glucose and one part fructose. So ... from glucose it came and unto glucose it shall return — once it hits your digestive system. The same is true for all naturally occurring sugars, with the exception of lactose. As it happens, lactose breaks down into glucose and an "odd duck" simple sugar, galactose (which I used to think was something in our solar system until I became a health writer). Just think of lactose as the "Milky Way" and you'll probably remember.

Simple sugars can get pretty complicated when you discuss their molecular structures. For example, simple sugars can be classified as monosaccharides (a.k.a. "single sugars") or disaccharides (a.k.a. "double sugars"). But unless you're writing a chemistry exam on sugars, you don't need to know this confusing stuff: you just need to know that all naturally occurring sugars wind up as glucose once you eat them. Glucose is carried to your cells through the bloodstream and is used as body fuel or energy.

How long does it take for a simple sugar to return to glucose? Well, it greatly depends on the amount of fiber in your food, how much protein you've eaten, and how much fat accompanies the sugar in your meal. If you have enough energy or fuel, once that sugar becomes glucose it can be stored as fat. And that's how — and why — sugar can make you fat.

What you have to watch out for is *added sugar* — sugar that manufacturers add to foods during processing or packaging. Foods containing fruit juice concentrates, invert sugar, regular corn syrup, honey, molasses, hydrolyzed lactose syrup, or high-fructose corn syrup (made out of highly concentrated fructose through the hydrolysis of starch), all have added sugars. Many people don't realize, however, that pure, *unsweetened* fruit juice is still a potent source of sugar, even when it contains no added sugar. Extra lactose (naturally occurring sugar in milk products), dextrose ("edible glucose"), and maltose (naturally occurring sugar in grains) are also contained in many of your foods. In other words, the products may have naturally occurring sugars anyway, and then *more* sugar is thrown in to enhance consistency, taste, and so on. The best way to know how much sugar is in a product is to look at the nutritional label for "carbohydrates."

What You Should Know about Sodium

Why cut down on sodium? To cut down on bloat. The more salt you eat, the more thirsty you get, and the more fluids you'll drink. If you cut the salt, you'll cut the thirst ... and the bloat. Your body will retain fluids when you've eaten a lot of salt to retain the right ratio of water to salt (that's your kidneys' job). The recommended nutrient intake (RNI) for sodium is 2,400 mg/day. But that is the *maximum* intake recommended, so anything less than that is even better.

To cut down on sodium, limit your salt intake to about 1-1/2 teaspoons per day. Cut out all foods high in sodium, such as canned soups, pickles, or soy sauce. (For example, some canned soups have sodium content as high as 1,000 mg, which is very high.) Look for labels that say the product is sodium-free or salt-free (this means there is no more than 5 mg of sodium for every 100-gram serving), or that it has low-sodium (this means 50 percent less sodium than the regular product and no more than 40 milligrams of sodium per 100-gram serving, with no *extra* salt added. "No salt added," or "unsalted" means just that — no salt has been added to the product.

Quitting Smoking

One of the best ways to reduce PMS severity is to quit smoking, since smoking greatly increases irritability, raises heart rate, increases blood pressure, and does all kinds of nasty things to your body! On the other hand, quitting smoking can greatly increase anxiety because of nicotine withdrawal. The symptoms of nicotine withdrawal begin within a few hours and peak at 24 to 48 hours after quitting. You may experience anxiety, irritability, hostility, restlessness, insomnia, and anger. For these reasons, many smokers turn to smoking cessation programs, which can include some of the following.

Herbal and Homeopathic Smoking Cessation Aids.
Many herbal and homeopathic smoking cessation products are available. Some use plant sources to reduce cravings; some work by using natural substances to help you "detox." For a list of natural smoking cessation products available in Canada, contact Canada's leading natural pharmacy, Smith's Pharmacy, at 1-800-361-6624 or visit **www.smithspharmacy.com**.

Behavioral Counseling.
Behavioral counseling, either in a group or individually, can raise the rate of abstinence to 20 to 25 percent. This approach to smoking cessation aims to change the mental processes of smoking, reinforce the benefits of nonsmoking, and teach skills to help the smoker avoid the urge to smoke.

Nicotine Gum.
Nicotine gum (Nicorette) is now available over the counter. It works as an aid to help you quit smoking by reducing nicotine cravings and withdrawal symptoms. Nicotine gum helps you wean yourself from nicotine by allowing you to gradually decrease the dosage until you stop using it altogether, a process that usually takes about 12 weeks.

The only disadvantage with this method is that it caters to the oral and addictive aspects of smoking (that is, rewarding the "urge" to smoke with a dose of nicotine).

Nicotine Patch.

Transdermal nicotine (Habitrol, Nicoderm, Nicotrol), or the "patch," doubles abstinence rates in former smokers. Most brands are now available over the counter. Each morning, a new patch is applied to a different area of dry, clean, hairless skin and left on for the day. Some patches are designed to be worn a full 24 hours. However, the constant supply of nicotine to the bloodstream sometimes causes very vivid or disturbing dreams. You can also expect to feel a mild itching, burning, or tingling at the site of the patch when it is first applied. The nicotine patch works best when it is worn for at least 7 to 12 weeks, with a gradual decrease in strength (i.e., nicotine). Many smokers find it effective because it allows them to tackle the psychological addiction to smoking before they are forced to deal with physical symptoms of withdrawal.

Nicotine Inhaler.

The nicotine inhaler (Nicotrol inhaler) delivers nicotine orally via inhalation from a plastic tube. Its success rate is about 28 percent, similar to that of nicotine gum. It's available by prescription only in the United States and has yet to make its debut in Canada. Like nicotine gum, the inhaler mimics smoking behavior by responding to each craving or "urge" to smoke, a feature that has both advantages and disadvantages to the smoker who wants to get over the physical symptoms of withdrawal. The nicotine inhaler should be used for a period of 12 weeks.

Nicotine Nasal Spray.

Like nicotine gum and the nicotine patch, nicotine nasal spray reduces craving and withdrawal symptoms, allowing smokers to cut back gradually. One squirt delivers about 1 mg nicotine. In three clinical trials involving 730 patients, 31 to 35 percent were still not smoking at six months. This compares to an average of 12 to 15 percent of smokers who were able to quit unaided. The nasal spray has a couple of advantages over the gum and the patch: nicotine is rapidly absorbed across the nasal membranes, providing a kick that is more like the real thing, and the prompt onset of action plus a flexible dosing schedule benefits heavier smokers. Because the nicotine reaches your bloodstream so quickly, nasal sprays do have a greater potential for addiction than the slower-acting gum and patch. Nasal sprays are not yet available for use in Canada.

Alternative Therapies.

Hypnosis, meditation, and acupuncture have helped some smokers quit. In the case of hypnosis and meditation, sessions may be private or part of a group smoking cessation program.

Eliminating Stress Hormones

Relieving stress comes from releasing stress hormones. One of the best ways to do this is through a good cry. Human tears contain high levels of stress hormone, which is one reason why people who cry tend to have less stress than those who do not cry. A dramatic movie can often induce tears, hence the term "tearjerker." They can serve an important purpose if you feel you need a good cry.

Laughter is another way of releasing stress because it makes us feel good, boosting endorphin levels in our bodies — which combat stress hormones. Laughter also causes deep muscle relaxation (which is why you can sometimes lose bladder control). Our blood pressure also drops, while the T-cells in our immune system increase. Incorporating humor into your life can be fun, too. Look for humorous books, magazines, or other materials and keep them handy. Get yourself onto a humor listserv, rent funny videos, watch comedy shows on TV, and use laughter to diffuse stress at the office or at home. Laughter bonds people and also attracts people to you. Teachers, doctors, or salespeople who generate laughter have more loyal students, more compliant patients, and higher sales!

Another great stress-reliever is forgiveness. When you have unresolved conflict with someone, or you're nursing a grudge, the emotional weight you carry when you think about the conflict increases blood pressure, stress hormones, heart rate, perspiration, and muscle tenseness. Forgiveness doesn't mean excusing bad behavior, but it does mean that you are prepared to move forward and let go of your bitterness toward that person. Forgiveness is healthier for you, and, chances are, the person with whom you are engaged in conflict would either welcome your forgiveness or, if also nursing a grudge, would, deep down, want to forgive you, too.

Forgiveness is about saying the "serenity prayer" (accepting the things you cannot change; changing the things you can). You can't change the fact that the conflict occurred, but you can change your current response to that conflict. Other things you cannot change include

- Other people
- Your age
- The way you were raised
- A death, illness, or accident in the family
- Being laid off from a job

   You *can* change

- Your reaction to others

- Your goals
- Your self-esteem and sense of self-worth
- How you treat others
- How you treat yourself
- Communicating your needs to others

Battling the Bloat

Premenstrual abdominal bloat and constipation, which can contribute to weight gain, are common premenstrual discomforts. I don't mean to sound like your mother, but are you eating enough fiber? Or the right kind, for that matter?

Fiber is the part of a plant your body can't digest, which comes in the form of both water-soluble fiber (which dissolves in water) and water insoluble fiber (which does not dissolve in water but, instead, absorbs water). Soluble and insoluble fiber differ, but they are equally beneficial.

Soluble fiber lowers the "bad" cholesterol, or low-density lipids (LDL), in your body. Experts aren't entirely sure how soluble fiber works its magic, but one popular theory is that it gets mixed into the bile the liver secretes and forms a type of gel that traps the building blocks of cholesterol, thus lowering your LDL levels. It's akin to a spider web trapping smaller insects

Insoluble fiber doesn't affect your cholesterol levels at all, *but it regulates your bowel movements*. How does it do this? As the insoluble fiber moves through your digestive tract, it absorbs water like a sponge and helps to transform your waste into a solid form faster, making the stools larger, softer, and easier to pass. Without insoluble fiber, your solid waste gets pushed down to the colon or lower intestine as always, but once there it is stored and dries out until you're ready to have a bowel movement. High-starch foods are associated with drier stools. This is exacerbated when you "ignore the urge," as the colon will dehydrate the waste even more until it becomes harder and difficult to pass, a condition known as constipation. Insoluble fiber will help to regulate your bowel movements by speeding things along. Insoluble fiber increases the "transit time" by increasing colon motility and limiting the time dietary toxins "hang around" the intestinal wall. This is why fiber can dramatically decrease your risk of colon cancer.

Sources of Insoluble Fiber

Good sources of insoluble fiber are wheat bran and whole grains, skins from various fruits and vegetables, seeds, leafy greens, and cruciferous vegetables (cauliflower, broccoli, brussels sprouts). The problem with grains is understanding what is truly "whole grain." For example, there is an assumption that because bread is dark or brown, it's more nutritious; this isn't necessarily so. In fact, many brown breads are simply made with enriched white flour and dyed with molasses. ("Enriched" means that nutrients lost during processing have been replaced.) High-fiber pita breads and bagels are available, but you have to search for them. A good rule is to simply look for the phrase "whole wheat," which means that the wheat is, indeed, whole.

Drink Water with Fiber

Think of fiber as a sponge. Obviously, a dry sponge won't work. You must soak it with water in order for it to be useful. Same thing here. Fiber without water is as useful as a dry sponge. *You gotta soak your fiber!* So here is the fiber/water recipe:

- Drink two glasses of water with your fiber. This means having a glass of water with whatever you're eating. Even if what you're eating does not contain much fiber, drinking water with your meal is a good habit to get into!
- Drink two glasses of water after you eat.

What about Vitamins and Minerals?

There is so much solid evidence on the benefits of vitamins and minerals in improving PMS that the American College of Obstetricians and Gynecologists (ACOG), in April 2001, revised its recommendations on PMS to include them. Keep in mind, though, that once you're eating more regularly, and eating the right balance of a variety of foods, you may not need further supplements. A lot of women who try taking vitamins and supplements without eating regularly may not benefit from vitamin supplements. Your blood sugar levels have to be stabilized first.

Vitamin B_6

Vitamin B_6 is an old standby that has raised some controversy. Most studies on vitamin B_6 conclude that up to 100 mg per day can improve PMS-related depression in particular. But at high doses, B_6 has disturbing side effects, known as neurotoxicity or nerve damage, which include pins and needles in the arms and legs, the feeling of an electric current running through the arms, surpersensitivity or burning of the skin, muscle weakness, numbness, shooting pains, and generalized itching. Some B_6 side effects can easily be mistaken for PMS: headaches, irritability, tiredness, depression, and puffy eyes. So please approach B_6 supplements with caution and do not exceed the 100-mg-per-day dosage.

Calcium

Consuming 1,200 to 1,500 mg of calcium daily has been shown in several clinical trials to significantly improve PMS. When progesterone receptors are blocked by low blood sugar levels or adrenaline, not enough progesterone can get to the cells, which means that important bone-building cells called osteoblasts are not being produced. This may explain why calcium supplements help ease PMS. In one study, women on calcium supplements for three months found that most of their PMS problems improved, with the exception of fatigue and insomnia.

Four glasses of milk are equal to about 1,200 mg of calcium. When you're trying to increase calcium in your diet, it also means avoiding foods that cause you to use up or "pee out" calcium, such as alcohol or coffee.

Maximizing Calcium Absorption

Calcium is best absorbed in an acidic environment. Do the following to increase acidity in your diet:

- Drink lemon juice in water with or after your meal.
- Add 2 tablespoons/30 mL apple cider vinegar and 2 tablespoons/30 mL raw honey or blackstrap molasses to 1 cup/250 mL water; drink with or after your meal.
- Use calcium-rich herbal vinegar in your salad dressing.

High-Calcium Sources

You may already know about some of these sources of calcium, but there may be some you aren't familiar with:

- Corn tortillas (Because these are made with lime, these are high in calcium.)
- Dandelion leaves
- Dried fruit (65 mg of calcium is in three small figs, a handful of raisins, four dates or eight prunes)
- Nettles
- Oats/oatmeal
- Sardines
- Seaweed

- Soy or tofu (not all tofu contains calcium; check labels)
- Tahini
- Yogurt

Calcium-Rich Greens.
Broccoli, kale, turnip greens, and mustard greens contain about 200 mg calcium. One cup cooked collards, wild onions, lamb's quarter, or amaranth greens contain about 400 mg calcium.

Calcium-Rich Herbs.
A big mug of infusion using any of these herbs is equal to 250 to 300 mg calcium. Add a big pinch of horsetail and increase the calcium by 10 percent.

- Nettle (*Urtica dioica*)
- Sage (*Salvia officinalis*)
- Chickweed (*Stellaria media*)
- Red clover (*Trifolium pratense*)
- Comfrey leaf (*Symphytum officinale*)
- Raspberry leaf (*Rubus species*)
- Oatstraw (*Avena sativa*)

The Uni-Tea Company makes a calcium-rich tea called FemininiTea that contains raspberry leaves, nettles, ginger, licorice, chamomile, sarsaparilla, rosemary, rose petals, yellow dock, uva ursi, Dong Quai, peony, lavender, and angelica. You can find this product in some health food or natural food stores.

Dairy Products.
The dairy product with the highest amount of calcium is live-culture yogurt (from milk without hormone and antibiotic residues). Yogurt also strengthens the digestive system, boosts the immune system, eases the nervous system, and helps prevent vaginal infections. Yogurt is much lower in fat than other dairy products, in case you want to stay heart healthy. In fact, 25 percent (350 to 400 mg) of your 1,500 mg daily calcium requirement can come from 1 cup/250 mL yogurt, which is equal to 1 cup/250 mL of milk, 1 ounce/30 grams hard cheese, or 1/2 cup/115 grams ricotta cheese. One cup of soy milk yields 80 mg calcium, and 1 cup almond milk yields 165 mg calcium.

Calcium Supplements.
If you can't get enough calcium in your diet, there are always supplements: 500 mg magnesium (not citrate) with calcium. Calcium supplements are more effective in

divided doses. Two doses of 250 mg, taken morning and night, actually provide more usable calcium than a 500 mg tablet. New research also shows that the amount of calcium absorbed from calcium citrate supplements is consistently higher than the amount absorbed from calcium carbonate supplements. Other popular sources of calcium supplements include

- Calcium-fortified orange juice (this is easier to digest and absorb then other supplements)
- Calcium citrate in tablet form (crushed tablets are better absorbed)
- Calcium gluconate, calcium lactate, and calcium carbonate (if chewable) — you can take 1,500 mg daily of one of these

Magnesium

Some studies show that small amounts of magnesium (no more than 200 mg/day) help to reduce water retention and bloating. Magnesium is found in leafy greens, seaweeds, nuts, whole grains, yogurt, cheese, potatoes, corn, peas, and squash. Herbal sources include oatstraw, licorice, kelp, nettle, dulse, burdock, chickweed, Althea root, horsetail, sage, raspberry leaf, red clover, valerian yellow dock, dandelion, carrot tops, parsley, and evening primrose.

Vitamin E

Some studies show that a dose of 400 IUs of vitamin E per day is useful in improving cramps and breast tenderness. To know which foods are a good source of vitamin E, the key word is *color*. Vitamin E is highest in non-green vegetables. The richer the color, the more E you get. Beets, carrots, and yams are all good sources. Vitamin E is also found in nuts, seeds, whole grains, fish-liver oils, freshly leafy greens, kale, cabbage, and asparagus. Otherwise, you can take a supplement. Herbal sources of vitamin E include alfalfa, rose hips, nettles, Dong Quai/Dang Gui, watercress, dandelions, seaweeds, and wild seeds.

Where to Find Your Vitamins and Minerals

Here's a summary of where you can find all the various nutrients you need to improve your mood and physical health (for magnesium, vitamin E, and calcium, see above):

Vitamin A/Beta-Carotene.
Vitamin A is found in liver, fish oils, egg yolks, whole milk, butter; beta-carotene (and A) is in leafy greens, yellow and orange vegetables, and fruits. Both are depleted by

coffee, alcohol, cortisone, mineral oil, fluorescent lights, liver "cleansing," excessive intake of iron, lack of protein.

Vitamin B_6.
Vitamin B_6 is found in meats, poultry, fish, nuts, liver, bananas, avocados, grapes, pears, egg yolk, whole grains, legumes.

Vitamin B_{12}.
Vitamin B_{12} is found in meats, dairy products, eggs, liver, fish. Both B_{12} and B_6 are depleted by coffee, alcohol, tobacco, sugar, raw oysters, and birth control pills.

Vitamin C.
Citrus fruits, broccoli, green pepper, strawberries, cabbage, tomato, cantaloupe, potatoes, and leafy greens contain vitamin C. Herbal sources include rose hips, yellow dock root, raspberry leaf, red clover, hops, nettles, pine needles, dandelion greens, alfalfa, echinacea, skullcap, parsley, cayenne, and paprika. Depleted by antibiotics, aspirin and other pain relievers, coffee, stress, aging, smoking, baking soda, and high fever.

Vitamin D.
Found in fortified milk, butter, leafy green vegetables, egg yolk, fish oils, butter, liver, skin exposure to sunlight, shrimp. Vitamin D is not found in plants, so there are no herbal sources. Depleted by mineral oil used on the skin, frequent baths, and sunscreens with SPF 8 or higher.

Vitamin K.
Found in leafy greens, corn and soybean oils, liver, cereals, dairy products, meats, fruits, egg yolk, blackstrap molasses. Herbal sources: nettles, alfalfa, kelp, green tea. Depleted by X-rays, radiation, air pollution, enemas, frozen foods, antibiotics, rancid fats, aspirin.

Thiamine (Vitamin B_1).
Found in asparagus, cauliflower, cabbage, kale, spirulina, seaweeds, citrus fruits. Herbal sources: peppermint, burdock, sage, yellow dock, alfalfa, red clover, fenugreek, raspberry leaves, nettles, catnip, watercress, yarrow, briar rose buds, and rose hips.

Riboflavin (Vitamin B_2).
Found in beans, greens, onions, seaweeds, spirulina, dairy products, mushrooms. Herbal sources: peppermint, alfalfa, parsley, echinacea, yellow dock, hops, dandelion, ginseng, dulse, kelp, fenugreek.

Pyridoxine (Vitamin B$_6$).

Found in baked potatoes with skin, broccoli, prunes, bananas, dried beans and lentils, all meats, poultry, and fish.

Folic Acid (B Factor).

Found in liver, eggs, leafy greens, yeast, legumes, whole grains, nuts, fruits (bananas, orange juice, grapefruit juice), vegetables (broccoli, spinach, asparagus, brussels sprouts). Herbal sources: nettles, alfalfa, parsley, sage, catnip, peppermint, plantain, comfrey leaves, chickweed.

Niacin (B Factor).

Found in grains, meats, nuts, and especially asparagus, spirulina, cabbage, bee pollen. Herbal sources: hops, raspberry leaf, red clover, slippery elm, echinacea, licorice, rose hips, nettles, alfalfa, parsley.

Bioflavonoids.

Found in citrus pulp and rind. Herbal sources: buckwheat greens, blue green algae, elder berries, hawthorn fruits, rose hips, horsetail, shepherd's purse.

Carotenes.

Found in carrots, cabbage, winter squash, sweet potatoes, dark leafy greens, apricots, spirulina, seaweeds. Herbal sources: peppermint, yellow dock, uva ursi, parsley, alfalfa, raspberry leaves, nettles, dandelion greens, kelp, green onions, violet leaves, cayenne, paprika, lamb's quarters, sage peppermint, chickweed, horsetail, black cohosh, rose hips.

Essential Fatty Acids (EFAs).

Essential fatty acids, including GLA, omega-6, and omega-3, are found in safflower oil and wheat germ oil. Herbal sources: all wild plants contain EFAs, especially evening primrose oil. Commercial sources: flax seed oil, evening primrose, black current, and borage.

Boron.

Found in organic fruits, vegetables, nuts. Herbal sources: all organic weeds including chickweed, purslane, nettles, dandelion, yellow dock.

Chromium.

Found in barley grass, bee pollen, prunes, nuts, mushrooms, liver, beets, whole wheat. Herbal sources: oatstraw, nettles, red clover, catnip, dulse, wild yam, yarrow, horsetail, black cohosh, licorice, echinacea, valerian, sarsaparilla. Depleted by white sugar.

Copper.
Found in liver, shellfish, nuts, legumes, water, organically grown grains, leafy greens, seaweeds, bittersweet chocolate. Herbal sources: skullcap, sage, horsetail, chickweed.

Iron.
Heme iron is easily absorbed by the body; non-heme iron not as easily absorbed, so should be taken with Vitamin C. Heme iron is found in liver, meat, and poultry; non-heme iron is found in dried fruit, seeds, almonds, cashews, enriched and whole grains, legumes, green leafy vegetables. Herbal sources: chickweed, kelp, burdock, catnip, horsetail, Althea root, milk thistle seed, uva ursi, dandelion leaf/root, yellow dock root, Dong Quai/Dang Gui, black cohosh, echinacea, plantain leaves, sarsaparilla, nettles, peppermint, licorice, valerian, fenugreek. Depleted by coffee, black tea, enemas, alcohol, aspirin, carbonated drinks, lack of protein, too many dairy products.

Manganese.
Found in any leaf or seed from a plant grown in healthy soil and found in seaweeds. Herbal sources: raspberry leaf, uva ursi, chickweed, milk thistle, yellow dock, ginseng, wild yam, hops, catnip, echinacea, horsetail, kelp, nettles, dandelion.

Molybdenum.
Found in organically raised dairy products, legumes, grains, leafy greens. Herbal sources: nettles, dandelion greens, sage, oatstraw, fenugreek, raspberry leaves, red clover, horsetail, chickweed, seaweeds.

Nickel.
Found in chocolate, nuts, dried beans, cereals. Herbal sources: alfalfa, red clover, oatstraw, fenugreek.

Phosphorus.
Found in whole grains, seeds, nuts. Herbal sources: peppermint, yellow dock, milk thistle, fennel, hops, chickweed, nettles, dandelion, parsley, dulse, red clover. Depleted by antacids.

Potassium.
Found in bananas, celery, cabbage, peas, parsley, broccoli, peppers, carrots, potato skins, eggplant, whole grains, pears, citrus, seaweeds. Herbal sources: sage, catnip, hops, dulse, peppermint, skullcap, kelp, red clover, horsetail, nettles, borage, plantain. Depleted by coffee, sugar, salt, alcohol, enemas, vomiting, diarrhea, chemical diuretics, dieting.

Selenium.

Found in dairy products, seaweeds, grains, garlic, liver, kidneys, fish, shellfish. Herbal sources: catnip, milk thistle, valerian, dulse, black cohosh, ginseng, uva ursi, hops, echinacea, kelp, raspberry leaf, rose buds and hips, hawthorn berries, fenugreek, sarsaparilla, yellow dock.

Silicon.

Found in unrefined grains, root vegetables, spinach, leeks. Herbal sources: horsetail, dulse, echinacea, cornsilk, burdock, oatstraw, licorice, chickweed, uva ursi, sarsaparilla.

Sulfur.

Found in eggs, dairy products, cabbage family plants, onions, garlic, parsley, watercress. Herbal sources: nettles, sage, plantain, horsetail.

Zinc.

Found in oysters, seafood, meat, liver, eggs, whole grains, wheat germ, pumpkin seeds, spirulina. Herbal sources: skullcap, sage, wild yam, chickweed, echinacea, nettles, dulse, milk thistle, sarsaparilla. Depleted by alcohol and air pollution.

When to Supplement

Supplementing your diet with a few of the following nutrients can help reduce your stress, and may dramatically improve PMS. When we're under stress, we're usually depleted in vitamins and minerals. Most of us know that the "anti-stress" vitamins are C (RNI is 4–8 g) and the B vitamins, particularly B_{12} (RNI is 50–250 mcg); niacin, or B_3 (RDI is 50–150 mg); B_6 (RNI is 50–100 mg.); and riboflavin, or B_2 (RNI is 50–100 mg). All of the B vitamins can be found in a B-complex vitamin supplement. But you should also supplement with the some of following (listed alphabetically). To avoid over- or under-supplementing (which can be affected by your diet), consult a doctor, nutritionist, or pharmacist about how much of the following to take:

- Beta-carotene
- Bioflavonoids
- Biotin
- Calcium
- Chromium
- Copper

- Folic acid
- Inositol
- Iodine
- Iron
- L-amino acids (e.g., L-glutamine; L-tyrosine; L-phenylalanine; and L-tryptophan)
- L-cysteine (take with vitamin C)
- Magnesium (an Epsom salt bath also contains magnesium)
- Manganese
- Molybdenum
- PABA
- Pancreatic enzymes (after meals)
- Pantothenic acid (B$_5$)
- Potassium
- Pyridoxal-5-phosphate
- Selenium
- Sulfur
- Superoxide dismutase (enzyme)
- Thiamine (B$_1$)
- Vitamin A
- Vitamin D
- Vitamin E
- Vitamin K
- Water (at least 2–3 quarts/liters per day)
- Zinc

Eating Disorders and PMS

For a significant percentage of the female population in North America, starving and purging are considered a normal way to control weight. Obviously, this wreaks havoc on your blood sugar levels, not to mention every organ in your body. In Western society, the fear of obesity is so crippling that 60 percent of young girls develop distorted body images between grades one and six, believing that they are "fat"; 70 percent of all women begin dieting between the ages of 14 and 21. A U.S. study of high-school girls found that 53 percent were unhappy with their bodies by age 13; and by age 18, 78 percent were dissatisfied. Eating disorders are so widespread that abnormal patterns of eating are increasingly accepted in the general population.

The two most common eating disorders involve starvation. They are *anorexia nervosa* ("loss of appetite due to mental disorder") and bingeing followed by purging, known as *bulimia nervosa* ("hunger like an ox due to mental disorder"). Women with bulimia nervosa purge after a bingeing episode by inducing vomiting or by abusing laxatives, diuretics, and thyroid hormone.

Perhaps the most accepted weight-control behavior is overexercising, which can affect your cycles (see Chapter 2, "Cycle-Logical Matters"). Today, rigorous, strenuous exercise is used as a method of "purging" and has become one of the tenets of socially accepted feminine behavior in our culture. A skeleton with biceps is the current ideal.

Women with a history of eating disorders, or who are practicing abnormal eating behaviors, are malnourished in all of the nutrients discussed in the previous section, but are particularly malnourished in calcium. They are at greater risk of osteoporosis after menopause, but may be suffering from more severe PMS as a result of calcium deficiency, too.

A small percentage of women suffer from a physical disorder called achalasia, in which muscles in the gastrointestinal tract do not relax, which can cause vomiting or reflux. If you suffer from this problem, you can be diagnosed with an eating disorder, such as bulimia, instead. Insist on a full gastrointestinal workup if you fall into this category. There are good medications that can help.

Physical Complications of Starving and Purging

If you have been starving, eating properly isn't easy, as the muscles in your gastrointestinal tract may not be working properly. Starvation causes them to slow down. As a result, you may feel full after eating a few bites and suffer from abdominal fullness and bloating, gas, nausea, and possibly heartburn from poor functioning of the lower esophageal sphincter. Constipation is another common problem experienced by recovering anorexics, caused by starvation. When your gastrointestinal tract slows down in the upper region, causing the fullness and bloating, it also slows down in the lower region, delaying the passage of stools. It's important to keep in mind that you may think you're constipated when you're simply experiencing a perfectly normal bowel pattern. For instance, when you're in the process of "refeeding" and just beginning to eat normally, it may take about a week for your body to pass stool, as it's busy taking in nutrients from your food.

When you binge, regardless of the "purge" method used, the binge episode by itself can cause symptoms such as abdominal bloating, distention, and fullness to the extent where breathlessness can occur, as your distended stomach presses up against your diaphragm. There are even documented cases of people requiring emergency surgery as a result of tears in the stomach wall, due to overstretching. The bingeing, of course, can also cause you to gain weight.

There are also complications from chronic self-induced vomiting, which means you self-induce vomiting one to three times per week or more. Problems that can complicate eating properly include super sensitivity in the mouth, caused by large amounts of stomach acid that are in vomit eroding the enamel off your teeth; swelling of the parotid gland, known as *sialadenosis*, which can give you "chipmunk" cheeks; chronic heartburn or "sour stomach"; and difficulty swallowing (known as *dysphagia*). You may also be dehydrated from the loss of electrolytes and fluids, and you'll need to drink plenty of water.

Compulsive Eating Disorders

When we hear "eating disorder," we usually think about anorexia or bulimia. There are many people, however, who binge without purging. This is also known as binge eating disorder (a.k.a. compulsive overeating), which has the one physical complication of weight gain and obesity, leading to problems with blood sugar control and insulin as well as a worsening of many PMS discomforts. In this case, the bingeing is still an announcement to the world that "I'm out of control." Someone who purges after bingeing is hiding a lack of control. Someone who binges and never purges is *advertising* his or her lack of control. The purger is passively asking for help; the binger who doesn't purge is aggressively asking for help. It's the same disease with a different result.

But there is one other factor when it comes to compulsive overeating, which is considered to be controversial and is often rejected by the overeater: the desire to get fat is often behind the compulsion. Many people who overeat insist that fat is a consequence of eating food, not a *goal*. Many therapists who deal with overeating disagree and believe that if a woman admits that she has an emotional interest in actually being large, she may be much closer to stopping her compulsion to eat. Furthermore, many women who eat compulsively do not recognize that they are doing so.

The following is a profile of a typical compulsive eater:

- Eating when you're not hungry
- Feeling out of control when you're around food, either trying to resist it or gorging on it
- Spending a lot of time thinking/worrying about food and your weight
- Always desperate to try another diet that promises results
- Feelings of self-loathing and shame
- Hating your own body
- Obsessed with what you can or will eat, or *have* eaten
- Eating in secret or with "eating friends"
- Appearing to be a professional dieter who's in control
- Buying cakes or pies as "gifts" and having them wrapped to hide the fact that they're for you
- Having a "pristine" kitchen with only the "right" foods
- Feeling either out of control with food (compulsive eating) or imprisoned by it (dieting)
- Feeling temporary relief by "not eating"
- Looking forward with pleasure and anticipation to the time when you can eat alone
- Feeling unhappy because of your eating behavior

The Issue of Hunger

Most people eat when they're hungry. But if you're a compulsive eater, hunger cues have nothing to do with when you eat. You may eat for any of the following reasons:

- At a social event, including family meals or meeting friends at restaurants. The point is that you plan food as the "social entertainment." Most of us do this, but often we do it when we're not even hungry.
- To satisfy "mouth hunger" — the need to have something in your mouth, even though you are not hungry.
- Eating to prevent *future* hunger: "Better eat now because later, I may not get a chance."
- Eating as a reward for a bad day or bad experience; or to reward yourself for a *good* day or good experience.
- Eating because "It's the only pleasure I can count on!"

- Eating to quell nerves.

- Eating because you're bored.

- Eating now because you're "going on a diet" tomorrow (hence, the eating is done out of a real fear that you will be deprived later).

- Eating because food is your friend.

12 Steps to Change

Food addiction, like other addictions, can be treated successfully with a 12-step program. For those of you who aren't familiar with this type of program, I've provided the text of "The 12 Steps" for overeaters in a box on the next page.

The 12-step program was started in the 1930s by an alcoholic, who was able to overcome his addiction essentially by saying, "God, help me!" He found other alcoholics who were in a similar position and through an organized, nonjudgmental support system, they overcame their addiction by realizing that "God" (a higher power, spirit, force, physical properties of the universe, or intelligence) *helps those who help themselves.* In other words, you have to want the help. This is the premise of Alcoholics Anonymous—the most successful recovery program for addicts that exists.

People with other addictions have adopted the same program, using "The 12 Steps and 12 Traditions," the founding literature for Alcoholics Anonymous. Overeaters Anonymous substitutes the phrase "compulsive overeater" for "alcoholic" and "food" for "alcohol." The theme of all 12-step programs is best expressed through the serenity prayer, the first line of which is "God grant me the serenity to accept the things I cannot change, courage to change the things I can, and the wisdom to know the difference." In other words, you can't take back the food you ate yesterday or last year; but you can control the food you eat today instead of feeling guilty about yesterday.

Every 12-step program also has the 12 traditions, which essentially is a code of conduct. To join an OA program, you need only to take the first step. Abstinence and the next two steps are what most people are able to do in 6 to 12 months before moving on. In an OA program, "abstinence" means three meals daily, weighed and measured, with nothing in between except sugar-free or no-calorie beverages and sugar-free gum. The food you eat is written down and called in. The program also advises you to get your doctor's approval before starting. Abstinence is continued through a continuous process that involves one day at a time and "sponsors" —

The 12 Steps of Overeaters Anonymous

Step One: I admit I am powerless over food and that my life has become unmanageable.

Step Two: I've come to believe that a Power greater than myself can restore me to sanity.

Step Three: I've made a decision to turn my will and my life over to the care of a Higher Power, as I understand it.

Step Four: I've made a searching and fearless moral inventory of myself.

Step Five: I've admitted to a Higher Power, to myself, and to another human being.

Step Six: I'm entirely ready to have a Higher Power remove all these defects of character.

Step Seven: I've humbly asked a Higher Power to remove my shortcomings.

Step Eight: I've made a list of all persons I have harmed and have become willing to make amends to them all.

Step Nine: I've made direct amends to such people wherever possible, except when to do so would injure them or others.

Step Ten: I've continued to take personal inventory and when I was wrong, promptly admitted it.

Step Eleven: I've sought through prayer and meditation to improve my conscious contact with a Higher Power, as I understand it, praying only for knowledge of Its will for me and the power to carry that out.

Step Twelve: Having had a spiritual awakening as the result of these steps, I've tried to carry this message to compulsive overeaters and to practice these principles in all my affairs.

Source: *Overeater's Anonymous*, 1997.

people who call you to check in and whom you can call when the cravings hit. Sponsors are recovering overeaters who have been there and who can talk you through your cravings.

OA membership is predominantly female. Many women overeat because they have been harmed by men, and their anger could be directed at any men in the room. This may not be a comfortable position for male overeaters. For this reason, OA is divided into all-female and all-male groups.

Exercise, the Outdoors, and PMS

Getting outdoors and exposing yourself to some real sunlight is the first step in combating PMS-related depression or low moods. Fifteen minutes of sunlight on your uncovered eyelids daily is the usual recommendation.

Aerobic exercise produces endorphins, "feel-good" hormones, which have been shown to decrease the incidence of depression. If you can't find the time or inclination to exercise, try to incorporate some activity into your day. Inactivity and sedentary living breeds depression and sadness. When you get up and do something, or see people, you feel more alive and part of this world.

Another important reason for exercise is to combat weight gain, which often occurs with depression, as you may turn to food for comfort. The more weight you gain, the more depressed you can feel, which fuels more comfort eating, and a worsening of depression.

The Benefits of Aerobic Exercise

All that jumping around and fast movement in aerobic exercise is done to create faster breathing so we can take in more oxygen into our bodies. How are we doing this? The blood contains oxygen! The faster your blood flows, the more oxygen can flow to your organs. When more oxygen is in our bodies, we burn fat, our blood pressure goes down, and our hearts work better. More oxygen also makes our brains work better, so we feel better. Studies show that depression is decreased when we increase oxygen flow into our bodies. Ancient techniques such as yoga, which specifically improve mental and spiritual well-being, achieve this in a different way by combining deep breathing and stretching, which improves oxygen and blood flow to specific parts of the body.

You can increase the flow of oxygen into your bloodstream without exercising your heart muscle by learning how to breathe deeply through your diaphragm. Many yoga-like programs and videos are available that can teach you this technique, which does not require you to jump around. The benefit is that you would be increasing the oxygen flow into your bloodstream, which is better than doing nothing at all to improve your health and has many health benefits, according to myriad wellness practitioners.

Active Living

If you don't exercise regularly, you can improve your health and well-being simply by leading a more active lifestyle. Here are some suggestions:

- If you drive everywhere, pick a parking space further away from your destination so you can work some daily walking into your life.
- If you take public transit everywhere, get off one or two stops early so you can walk the rest of the way to your destination.
- Choose stairs more often than escalators or elevators.
- Park at the one side of the mall and then walk to the other.
- Take a stroll around your neighborhood after dinner.
- Volunteer to walk the dog.
- On weekends, go to the zoo, the park, or out to flea markets, and so on.

Looking into Yoga

Yoga does not consist of just various stretches or postures, but is actually a way of life for many. It is part of a whole science of living known as Ayurveda (see Chapter 5). Practicing yoga is a preventative health science that involves certain physical postures, exercises, and meditation. Essentially, yoga is the "exercise" component of Ayurveda. It involves relaxing meditation, breathing, and physical postures designed to tone and soothe your mental and physical state. Most people benefit from introductory yoga classes, or even from introductory videos.

Deep-Breathing Exercises

Deep breathing helps to relieve a range of PMS-related symptoms such as anxiety and irritability. In fact, sighing and yawning are signs that you're not getting enough oxygen in your body; the sigh or yawn is your body's way of righting the situation. The following deep breathing techniques are modeled after yogic breathing exercises. Deep breathing calms the nervous system, relaxes the small arteries, and permanently lowers blood pressure.

Abdominal Breathing.
Lie down on a mat or on your bed. Take slow, deep, rhythmic breaths through your nose. When your abdominal cavity is expanded, it means the your lungs have filled completely, which is important. Then, slowly exhale completely, watching your abdomen collapse again. Repeat 6 to 10 times. Practice this morning and night.

Extended Abdominal Breathing.
This is a variation on the above. When your abdomen expands with air, try three more short inhalations. It's akin to adding those last drops of gas in your tank when

your tank is full. Then, when you exhale in one long breath, don't inhale yet. Take three more short exhales.

Abdominal Lift.
Stand with your feet at about shoulder width, bend your knees slightly, bend forward from the waist, exhale completely, and brace your hands above the knees. Then lift the abdomen upward while holding your exhalation. Your abdomen should look concave. Stand erect again and inhale just before you feel the urge to gasp. Greer Childers, in her video "Body Flex," demonstrates this technique very well.

Rapid Abdominal Breathing.
This is abdominal breathing done at a fast speed so it feels as though your inhalations and exhalations are forceful and powerful. Try this for 25 to 100 repetitions. Each breath should last only a second or so, compared to the 10 to 20 seconds involved in regular deep abdominal breathing.

Alternate Nostril Breathing.
Hold one nostril closed, inhaling and exhaling deeply. Then alternate nostrils. This is often done prior to meditation. Alternate nostril breathing is thought to balance the left and right sides of the brain.

Meditation as an Exercise

Meditation simply requires you to *stop thinking* (about your life, problems, etc.) and *just be*. To do this, people usually find a relaxing spot, sit quietly, and breathe deeply for a few minutes. Going for a nature walk, playing golf, listening to music, reading inspiring poetry or prose, gardening, listening to silence, and listening only to the sounds of your own breathing are all forms of meditation. The following are just a few activities that can be meditative:

- Taking a walk or hike
- Swimming
- Running or jogging
- Gardening
- Golfing
- Appreciating music (listening, dancing, etc.)
- Reading for pleasure
- Walking your dog
- Practicing breathing exercises

- Practicing stretching exercises
- Practicing yoga or Qi Gong

Stretching

Why do cats stretch each time they get up? They have a natural desire to stretch because it improves muscle blood flow, oxygen flow, and digestion.

Postures and Stretches to Improve Tranquility

The following stretches will help relieve stress and improve tranquility.

- While sitting or standing, raise your arms above your head. Keep the shoulders relaxed and breathe deeply for five seconds. Release and repeat five times.

- Gently raise your shoulders in an exaggerated shrug. Breathe deeply and hold for 10 seconds. Relax, and repeat three times.

- Lotus: Sit cross-legged on the floor with spine straight and neck aligned. Focus on your breath, letting it gently fill the diaphragm and the back of the rib cage. On the inhalation, say "SO" and on the exhalation, say "HUM." Voicing the breath in this manner will keep you focused and relaxed. Continue with "SO-HUM" until you feel at ease.

- Child's Pose: Sit on your heels. Bring your forehead to the floor in front of you. Breathe into the back of the rib cage, feeling the stretch in your spine. Hold as long as it's comfortable.

- Tree: Stand tall and focus your gaze on a point across the room. Place the heel of one foot on the opposite inner thigh. Float your arms upward until your palms are touching. Breathe deeply, and hold for five seconds. Release and repeat on the other side.

- Savasana or "Corpse" Pose: Lie on your back with palms facing upward, feet turned gently outwards. Focus on the movement of breath throughout your body.

- Bow: Lie on your belly, with arms at your sides. Bend your legs at the knees and bring your heels in towards your buttocks. Reach back and take hold of the right, then the left ankle. Flex your feet if you're having a hard time maintaining this position. Inhale, raising the upper body as far off the floor as possible. Lift your head, completing the arch. Your knees should remain as close together as possible (tying them together might help here). Breathe deeply and hold for 10 to 15 seconds.

Try Qi Gong Exercises

Every morning, all over China, people of all ages gather at parks to do their daily Qi Gong exercises. Pronounced "Ch'i Kung," these are exercises that help get your life force energy (called *qi* or "chi" in Chinese) flowing and unblocked. Qi Gong exercises are modeled after movements in wildlife (such as birds or animals) and movement of trees and other things in nature. The exercises have a continuous flow, rather than the stillness of a posture seen in yoga. Using the hands in various positions to gather in the *qi*, move the *qi*, or release the *qi* is one of the most important aspects of Qi Gong movements.

One of the first group of Qi Gong exercises you might learn are the "seasons" – fall, winter, spring, summer, and late summer (there are five seasons here). These exercises look more like a dance, with precise, slow movements. The word *qi* means vitality, energy, and life force; the word *gong* means practice, cultivate, refine. The Chinese believe that practicing Qi Gong balances the body and improves physical and mental well-being. These exercises push the life force energy into the various meridian pathways that correspond to organs. It is the same map used in pressure-point healing. Qi Gong improves oxygen flow and enhances the lymphatic system. It is similar to Tai Chi, except it allows for greater flexibility in routine. The best place to learn Qi Gong is through a qualified instructor. You can generally find Qi Gong classes through the alternative healing community. Check health food stores and other centers that offer classes such as yoga or Tai Chi. Qi Gong is difficult to learn from a book or video. An instructor is best.

Exercising Your Mind

Creativity can dramatically lower stress levels, too, including art in all its forms: words, fine arts, visual arts, healing arts, performing arts, hobbies, or sport. Writing, in particular — in the form of keeping a journal or writing poetry or letters — is a stress-buster. A new study published in *The Journal of the American Medical Association* found that people suffering from chronic ailments such as asthma or arthritis actually felt better when they wrote about their ailments.

A few years ago, Oprah Winfrey used her influence to get her viewers to begin daily diary writing or "journaling" because of the powerful effects it can have on enabling those of us who are otherwise without voice or expression. Using *her* own creativity to enable others, she has "resold" the idea of keeping a journal in an age when few people take the time to sit down and be still with their thoughts. Oprah has taken journaling one step further by encouraging people to begin "gratitude journaling," where they think about what in their lives they are thankful for, and actually write it down. A firm believer in literacy as well, Oprah's influence on the comeback of journals can also enable many who, in the past, might have been afraid to write because of their education levels, to find the courage to write and express themselves. For women who do not feel they are "creative" or "artistic," keeping a journal is an opportunity for them to express their feelings and passions.

7

AN HERBAL AND
HANDS-ON APPROACH

One Native North American tribe believes that disease was given to humans by the animals in an effort to even out the odds for survival. Members of the plant kingdom had a meeting about this and decided that they would do their best to cure disease, making themselves available to man for preventative and curative remedies.

Every culture in the world has relied on plants and herbs to treat illness — including Western medicine. Herbal therapies were taken as early as 4000 B.C. by the Sumerians, 1,000 years before Chinese herbs were first used. By 3000 B.C., the Chinese were using over 1,000 medicinal herbs.

Much like the pharmaceutical drugs of today, herbal therapies became established through trial and error. The herbs available today in your health food stores and pharmacies are considered not just effective, but powerful enough to do harm if they are not taken properly. And 25 percent of all prescription drugs in North America are derived from plants, too. Herbal medicine is becoming so popular because people are realizing that, often, the over-the-counter or prescription drugs are no more or less potent. So why not go more natural?

North America is divided at the U.S. and Canadian border over how to classify herbs. Alternative medicine practitioners argue that pharmaceutical companies won't fund research into herbal therapies because these remedies are natural and hence, cannot be patented.

North Americans purchase a few billion dollars' of herbs and vitamins a year. And sales keep going up. Plant drugs are classified as "food" or "food additives" in the U.S., and therefore many herbs are sold in grocery stores, health food stores, or pharmacies. Canada allows the sale of drugs that have received a drug identification number — something that many herbs do not have. Herbs that cannot be found in pharmacies can be found in health food stores or Chinese herb stores (which large Canadian cities have in abundance). But a few natural products are actually banned in Canada, including melatonin.

This chapter explores how herbs can help improve premenstrual discomforts, with the exception of herbs that are good sources of calcium, which I discussed in Chapter 6, "The Diet and Exercise Approach." The most important herbal supplements for PMS are the "nerve herbs" — herbs that can calm you down and can help alleviate stress, which, in turn, can restore progesterone receptor functioning. As well, a variety of herbs can be used to help combat depression. Finally, some herbs can help control your cycle and alleviate specific physical discomforts, such as bloating.

A Word about the Placebo Effect

Herbs are often "pooh-poohed" by medical doctors as not well studied, or as being proven successful based on only anecdotal evidence. There has been a rash of studies comparing various herbs to placebos (fake pills), with often very conflicting results.

One of the best episodes of *M*A*S*H* revolved around the use of placebos in place of an effective painkiller. Desperate, and without a supply of painkillers for an unexpected influx of wounded, Hawkeye suggests to his colleagues that they try a placebo, and simply tell patients that they are being given a "very powerful drug" instead of a sugar pill. Despite the skeptical objections raised by his colleagues, Hawkeye wins again — *it works.* The patients' expectation and belief that they are receiving a powerful painkiller produces the "placebo effect" — a real, physical, analgesic effect.

This type of effect is why testing an herb against a placebo is not always reliable, according to critics of placebo-controlled trials. The fact that red placebo stimulants produce greater effects than blue, or that placebo injections are more effective than oral placebos, means that the placebo can be viewed as a separate and distinct pharmacological entity, with its own set of toxicity and side effects rather than "nothing" or "zero." So next time you read that a certain herb did not perform well compared to a placebo, look for the anecdotal evidence, too. It often counts for more.

When comparing an herb to a placebo, we are supposed to be answering the question, "Is this herb better than nothing?" But that's not what a placebo-controlled study answers. It answers whether the real biological effects of the herb, combined with the real biological effects of the "placebo effect," produce the desired results.

Another myth about placebo-controlled trials is that they are "blind." (In a blind trial, both the study participants and the dispensers of the pills do not know who is getting a dummy pill and who is getting the real pill.) Critics point out that placebo-controlled trials routinely become "unblinded" (people drop out of the trial or it becomes very clear who is getting the real herb or drug).

Flower Power for Cycle Control

Many women rely on traditional medicine to help regulate their cycles or cope with heavy flows. Regulating your cycle, one of the keys to reducing premenstrual discomforts, can be done through natural means, which include adjusting your diet and activity patterns (see Chapter 6, "The Diet and Exercise Approach" — often too much

TABLE 7.1   How to Make an Herbal Infusion

An infusion is a large amount of dried (not fresh) herb brewed for a long time. An infusion extracts more nutrients than a tincture (herb in a solution of alcohol) and more medicinal qualities than a tea (a small amount of fresh or dried herb brewed for a short time). Most infusions are short-lived; they're good for just two or three days.

Prepare infusions in pint/half-liter and quart/liter jars with tight lids. A teapot is not as good, but acceptable.

The usual dose of infusion is 1–2 cups a day, taken hot, chilled, or at room temperature. Infusions may be seasoned with sweeteners, tamari, milk, or any addition that pleases your taste. Infusions can be used as soup stocks, bath waters, hair rinses, facial washes, and so on.

Combine...	In...	For...
Roots/bark, 1 oz./30 g	1 pint/500 mL water	8 hours minimum
Leaves, 1 oz./30 g	1 quart/1 liter water	4 hours minimum
Flowers, 1 oz./30 gm	1 quart/1 liter water	2 hours maximum
Seeds/berries, 1 oz./30 g	1 quart/1 liter water	30 minutes maximum

Source: Adapted from Susun S. Weed, *Wise Women Ways: Menopausal Years.*

exercise does more damage than moderate exercise). If you're looking for specific remedies for irregular cycles and heavy flows, this is the place to be.

Irregular Cycles

It's been found that both regular orgasms (through partnered or self-stimulation) and pelvic floor exercises can help maintain regular periods. For irregular cycles, including amenorrhea, the following herbs are reportedly helpful. The Latin name for each herb is in brackets, although it may not be on the label of the herb.

- **Raspberry leaf** (*Rubus* species). Best as an infusion (see Table 7.1). Nourishes the ovaries as well as the uterus, helps with erratic periods.

- **Dong Quai/Dang Gui compound** (*Angelica sinensis*). As a tincture, this warms, regulates, and gently heals the entire reproductive system; especially useful if your irregular cycles are accompanied with premenstrual discomforts. (Note: Dong Quai can aggravate fibroids.)

- **Liferoot blossom** (*Senecio aureus*). Helps tone the reproductive hormones, ovaries, uterus, adrenals, liver, and pituitary gland. As a tincture, take five drops daily.

- **Chasteberry** (*Vitex agnus castus*). As a tincture, this helps with irregular periods. Use one "dropperful" in a small glass of water two or three times daily for six to eight weeks after every irregular period.

- **Cinnamon bark** (*Cinnamomum zeylanicum*). This invigorates the blood, helps regulate the menstrual cycle, and helps with very heavy flows as well, especially during perimenopause. Sip one cup/250 mL of infusion (see Table 7.1), use five to ten drops of tincture once or twice a day, gnaw on a cinnamon stick, or simply sprinkle cinnamon on everything.

Estrogen Herbs

The following herbs help promote estrogen production and stabilize infrequent periods, and may reduce the severity of estrogen-loss discomforts during perimenopause:

- Alfalfa (*Medicago sativa*) and red clover (*Trifolium pratense*) flowers and leaves
- Black cohosh root (*Cimicifuga racemosa*)
- Hops (*Humulus lupus*), female flowers
- Licorice root (*Glycyrrhiza glabra*)
- Sage leaves (*Salvia officinalis*)
- Sweet briar hips or leaf buds (*Rosa rubiginosa*)
- Pomegranate seeds
- Any herb containing flavonoids

Progesterone Herbs

The following herbs help promote progesterone production and help stabilize too-frequent periods, which can occur as you approach perimenopause:

- Chasteberry/vitex berries (*Vitex agnus castus*)
- Sarsaparilla roots (*Smilax* species)
- Wild yam roots (*Dioscorea villosa*)
- Yarrow flowers and leaves (*Achillea millefolium*)

For Heavy Flows

If you're coping with very heavy menstrual flows, it's important to consume roughly 2 mg iron from herbs or foods while the bleeding persists. This will help to prevent anemia. Iron is best in small doses throughout the day, rather than in one big gulp. Coffee, black tea, soy protein, egg yolks, bran, and calcium supplements over 250 mg can also impair iron absorption.

Bleeding can be aggravated by aspirin, Midol, and larger doses of ascorbic acid (vitamin C supplements) because they thin the blood. In general, foods rich in bioflavonoids and carotene (anything rich in color, such as carrots, beets, and tomatoes) will help with blood loss.

- Cinnamon bark (*Cinnamomum zeylanicum*). Instructions for how to take it can be found above, under "Irregular Cycles."
- Dandelion leaves are the best source of usable iron, containing roughly 30 grams of iron per ounce.
- Lady's mantle (*Alchemilla vulgaris*), the "alchemical weed," controlled heavy bleeding in virtually all of more than 300 women in a recent study.
- Wild yam root (*Dioscorea villosa*). As a tincture, 20–30 drops daily for the two weeks before your period can help reduce flow.
- Shepherd's purse (*Capsella bursa-pastoris*). Commonly used to stop bleeding or reduce flow. Available dried and as a liquid extract. Can cause heart palpitations in large doses and should not be taken with an anticoagulant.
- Yellow dock root (*Rumex crispus*). An alcohol- or vinegar-based tincture is best: 20 drops of alcohol-based tincture or 3 teaspoons/15 mL vinegar-based tincture, taken in tea or water, gives 1 mg iron to the blood.

These greens are high sources of iron: spinach, swiss chard (silver beet), beet greens, wood sorrel, and rhubarb.

For Menstrual Cramps

The following herbs are helpful in relieving cramps. Many of them have an anti-prostaglandin effect, which is why they work. (Prostaglandins are the chemicals that make you "squeeze" and contract.)

- Black yaw (*Viburnum prunifolium*)
- Blue cohosh (*Caulophyllum thalictroides*)
- Cinnamon
- Cloves
- Cramp bark (*Viburnum opulus*)
- Evening primrose (*Oenothera biennis*)
- False unicorn root (*Chamaelireum luteum*)
- Feverfew (*Tanacetum parthenium*)

- Flax seed (*Linum usitatissimum*)
- Garlic
- Ginger
- Hops (*Humulus lupus*)
- Meadowsweet (*Filipendula ulmaria*)
- Motherwort (*Leonurus cardiaca*)
- Red raspberry (*Rubus species*)
- Thyme
- Wild yam (*Dioscorea villosa*)
- Yarrow (*Achillea millefolium*)

The following oils are recommended to relieve cramps, in order of best known: clary sage (*Salvia sclarea*); cypress (*Cupressus sempervirens*); chamomile (Roman); geranium, jasmine, and lavender. Peppermint, sage, tarragon, and thyme are also recommended but are best applied to the soles of the feet, as they're very strong.

Herbs that Calm

Taking an herb is not going to change stressful or depressing circumstances that are occurring in your life. But they may help take the "edge" off in combination with counseling (see Chapter 3, "The Emotional Premenstrual Signs," for more on therapy). A variety of "nerve herbs" have exploded onto the marketplace over the last decade, which have been effective in treating mild to moderate depression, or which are known to improve your mood.

St. John's Wort

St. John's wort, also known as hypericum (from its Latin name, *Hypericum perforatum*), has been used as a sort of "nerve tonic" in folk medicine for centuries. It's been shown to successfully treat mild to moderate depression and anxiety. St. John's wort has been used in Germany for years as a first-line treatment for depression, and it is endorsed by the American Psychiatric Association. In Germany and other parts of Europe, it outsells Prozac prescriptions. In a preliminary study at the Department of Complementary Medicine of the University of Exeter in Britain, it was shown that using 300 mg of St. John's wort daily improved many PMS discomforts, while premenstrual mood-related changes were improved by 85 percent and crying was reduced by 92 percent.

Since it was introduced into North America in the early 1990s, millions of North Americans have been successfully treated for depression with St. John's wort. In the United States, sales of St. John's wort and other botanical products reached an estimated $4.3 billion dollars in 1998, according to *Nutrition Business Journal*.

The benefits of St. John's wort are that it has minimal side effects, it can be mixed with alcohol, it is nonaddictive, and you don't need to increase your dose over time as you do with antidepressants. You can go on and off of St. John's wort as you wish, without any problem; it helps you sleep and dream; and it doesn't have any sedative

Buyer Beware

Naturally (no pun intended!), since St. John's wort is so popular, many companies now make it. But recent studies show that not all brands of St. John's wort are equal — a hazard of a fast-growing herbal therapy market that has yet to set standards. The *Los Angeles Times* conducted a consumer study that revealed three out of ten brands of St. John's wort had no more than about half the potency listed on the label, while four other brands had less than 90 percent of the potency listed. Since Canadian guidelines for herbal products are in flux, we have to assume that there is some inequality of brands in Canada, too. If you're considering taking St. John's wort, ask health food store owners and pharmacists about recommended brands, and call the manufacturers of various brands for more information about processing and quality control. For now, there are no other ways to ensure quality other than using your consumer power to ask questions!

More generally, of the roughly 600 herbs available in the United States (fewer are available in Canada), fewer than 12 have been tested in scientifically controlled trials, which is the process that usually determines whether an herb is safe and works better than a placebo. About 50 herbs have been tested under more lax conditions.

Canadian labels will tell you what additives you're getting when you purchase a vitamin or supplement, such as yeast, sugar, or coloring. They will also tell you what that vitamin or supplement does not contain.

As of this writing, the American Herbal Products Association, which is a trade group of herbal manufactures, was compiling a reference manual on 600 herbal ingredients, including directions for safe use. Some experts suggest comparing most of the herbs sold to coffee when weighing "dosage": two cups of coffee per day is considered safe; five cups may cause headaches and nervousness; 15 cups can cause serious side effects. In other words, don't overconsume the herb. More isn't necessarily more effective.

effect — in fact, it enhances your alertness. And finally, it doesn't put you at risk for agitation or hypomania.

The downside of St. John's wort is that there is a longer lag time before you feel its effects compared to prescription antidepressants, which means that it may not work well in severe depression. It can also make you oversensitive to sunlight and may have some gastrointestinal side effects, such as nausea, loss of appetite, or abdominal pains. Experts advise that simply taking the herb with meals will alleviate the problem. Some people are allergic to St. John's wort and can develop skin rashes from taking it.

SAM-e

SAM-e, pronounced "Sammy," is another natural compound that has been shown to help alleviate depression in mild to moderate cases. Sam-e stands for S-adenosylmethionine, a compound made by your body's cells. Since it was introduced in the United States in March 1999, more people have purchased Sam-e than St. John's wort. One reason could be that Sam-e has been shown to help relieve joint pain and also improve liver function, which makes it popular for the people suffering from arthritis as well as depression.

Studies done in Italy during the 1970s documented SAM-e's effectiveness as an antidepressant; recent U.S. studies confirm the same results. Right now, psychiatrists are endorsing the use of SAM-e in cases of mild to moderate depression. But similar to the effects of antidepressants, some Sam-e users experience mild mania (see the section on antidepressants in Chapter 9, "Prescription Drugs used for PMS"). Some people have also reported hot, itchy ears as a side effect. Although SAM-e is available over the counter in Canada and the United States, it is still only available by prescription in Europe. If you're interested in trying SAM-e, discuss its availability with your family doctor.

Kava Root (a.k.a. Kava Kava)

From the black pepper family, another popular herb is kava (*Piper methysticum*), which has been a popular herbal drink in the South Pacific for centuries. Kava grows on the islands of Polynesia and is known to calm nerves and ease stress, fatigue, and anxiety, which results in an antidepressant effect. Kava can also help alleviate migraine headaches and menstrual cramps. Placebo-controlled studies conducted by the U.S. National Institute of Mental Health showed that kava significantly relieved anxiety and stress, without the problem of dependency or addiction to the herb.

Kava should not be combined with alcohol because it can make the effects of alcohol more potent. You should also check with your doctor before you combine kava with any prescription medications.

Other Mood Compounds

Some of the following are phytochemicals (food chemicals), but most are available as supplements over the counter. They can help combat depression, sleeplessness, and stress.

- **Gamma-aminobutyric acid (GABA).** This is an amino acid that is supposedly an antianxiety agent, which may also help you to fall asleep if you suffer from sleeplessness.
- **Inositol.** This is a naturally occurring antidepressant that is present in many foods, such as vegetables, whole grains, milk, and meat, and should be available over-the-counter.
- **Dehydroepiandrosterone (DHEA).** This is a hormone produced by the adrenal glands; production declines as we age. It has been shown to improve moods and memory in certain studies, but is not available yet in Canada.
- **Melatonin.** This is a hormone that improves sleep and helps reset the body's natural clock. It is not available in Canada.
- **Phosphatidylserine (PS).** This is a phospholipid, a substance that feeds brain-cell membranes. Some studies show it has natural antidepressant qualities.
- **Tetrahydrobiopterin (BH4).** This substance activates enzymes that control serotonin, norepinephrine, and dopamine levels, which are all important for stable moods. Some studies show BH4 is an effective natural treatment for depression.
- **Phenylethylamine (PEA).** This is a nitrogen-containing compound found in small quantities in the brain. Studies show it works as a natural antidepressant.
- **Rubidium.** Rubidium is a natural chemical in our bodies, belonging to the same family as lithium, potassium, and sodium. Studies show that it can work as an antidepressant.
- **Ginkgo.** This is a plant used to treat a variety of ailments and is a common herb in Chinese medicine. It can improve memory, and some studies show that it acts as an antidepressant.
- **Valerian root** (*Valeriana officinalis*). This is similar to kava root in that it works as an antianxiety agent, as well as combating insomnia. The only problem with

valerian root is the smell: it really smells bad, so be sure to seal it in an airtight container.

Consider Aromatherapy

Essential oils, made from plants (mostly herbs and flowers), can do wonders to relieve stress naturally; many essential oils are known for their calming and antidepressant effects. The following essential oils are known to have calming, sedative, and/or antidepressant effects: ylang-ylang, jasmine, neroli (a.k.a. orange blossom), cedar, lavender (a few drops on your pillow will also help you sleep), chamomile, marjoram, geranium, patchouli, rose, sage, clary sage, and sandalwood.

In general, the following essential oils are considered "essential" for the female system, in terms of balancing hormones and offsetting a number of PMS discomforts: bergamot, clary sage, clove, fennel, geranium, nutmeg, sage, and ylang-ylang. See Table 7.2 for specific complaints. All the oils listed can be used in a diffuser (a ceramic pot with a tea light underneath and a bowl of water on top into which the oils are dropped; a light bulb ring also works); in a hot bath (you can drop the oils directly into the hot water); or as a massage oil (you need a "carrier" base oil such as olive, jojoba, carrot-seed, grapeseed, or sweet-almond). You can also mix certain oils into an unscented moisturizer and apply to your face (neroli, lavender, ylang-ylang, and rose all make excellent "facial oils). Twelve drops of oil in any of these methods is the average "dose." When oils are applied directly to the skin, two drops is the average amount to use. Applying any of the oils directly to the soles of the feet is a good way to feel the effectiveness faster.

The following scents are considered stimulating and energizing: lemon, grapefruit, peppermint, rosemary, and pine. See Table 7.2 for the full range of essential oils you can use to ease premenstrual discomforts, both emotional and physical.

Herbs That Relieve Physical Discomforts

The following are herbs that can be used to improve premenstrual physical discomforts, listed in alphabetical order.

- Alfalfa (*Medicago sativa*), for bloating
- Black cohosh (*Cimicifuga racemosa*), for joint pain, headaches, depression
- Chasteberry (*Vitex agnus castus*), for breast tenderness, anxiety, insomnia, mood swings
- Chickweed (*Stellaria media*), for bloating

- Dandelion, for bloating

- Evening primrose oil, for cramps, breast tenderness (see separate section)

- Ginger, for nausea

- Nettle (*Urtica dioica*), for bloating

- Uva ursi (also known as bearberry, *Arctostaphylos uva-ursi*), for bloating

TABLE 7.2 Aromatherapy for PMS

TO HELP WITH FEELINGS OF...	TRY...
Anger, rage, or anxiety	*Calming scents*: bergamot, cedarwood, chamomile, clary sage, geranium, jasmine, lavender, myrrh, neroli, patchouli, rose, sage, sandalwood, tangerine, ylang-ylang
Decreased concentration or confusion (extremely rare)	*Stimulating scents:* basil, cedarwood, cypress, fir, frankincense, geranium, ginger, jasmine, juniper, marjoram, peppermint, rose, rosemary, rosewood, sandalwood, spruce, thyme, ylang-ylang
Depression	See under *Anger;* also, to invigorate, try frankincense, ginger, grapefruit, juniper, pepper, and rosewood, for stimulation
Emotional overresponsiveness	See under *Anger*
Forgetfulness	Basil, bergamot, clove, ginger, grapefruit, lavender, lemon, cedarwood, chamomile (Roman), cypress, fir, geranium, juniper, marjoram, myrrh, orange, rose, rosemary, sandalwood, rose, ylang-ylang
Loss of control	See under *Anger*
Melancholy	See under *Anger*
Restlessness	Angelica, basil, bergamot, cedarwood, frankincense, geranium, lavender, orange, rose, rosewood, spruce, valor, ylang-ylang

TO HELP COMBAT...	TRY...
Abdominal bloating (which may also cause weight gain)	Cypress, fennel, juniper, geranium, lemongrass, rosemary, tangerine
Acne or other skin eruptions	Bergamot, cedarwood, chamomile, clary sage, eucalyptus, juniper, lavender, lemon, marjoram, tea tree oil, patchouli, rosemary, rosewood, sage, thyme (can be applied on the blotches directly)
Asthma	Cypress, eucalyptus, fir, frankincense, hyssop, lavender, lemon, marjoram, myrrh, myrtle, oregano, peppermint, ravensara, rose, rosemary, sage, thyme (can apply to pillow, or over lungs/throat topically)
Backache (e.g., low back pain)	As a massage oil: cypress, helichrysum, peppermint

TABLE 7.2 Aromatherapy for PMS (continued)

TO HELP COMBAT...	TRY...
Breast swelling and tenderness	Clary sage, cypress, fennel, geranium, lemongrass, sage, spearmint
Changes in sex drive (either more or less)	Geranium, jasmine, lavender, patchouli, rose, sandalwood, ylang-ylang (these are aphrodisiacs)
Chills, shakiness, and dizziness	Ginger (apply to bottoms of feet)
Clumsiness and poor coordination	Cedarwood, chamomile, frankincense, and ylang-ylang (promote a feeling of "balance" emotionally and physically)
Constipation	Fennel, ginger, juniper, marjoram, orange, patchouli, pepper (black), rose, rosemary, sandalwood, tangerine, tarragon (can be applied as a massage oil to the lower abdomen)
Diarrhea	Geranium, ginger, myrrh, myrtle, peppermint, sandalwood, spearmint, tea tree
Eye problems	Chamomile, cypress, fennel, frankincense, lavender, lemon, lemongrass. (Diffuse or bathe in these oils. Good for improving vision and promoting eyesight. *Do not drop in eyes or use around eyes.*)
Fatigue	Basil, clove, ravensara, rosemary, thyme
Headaches	Clove, eucalyptus, frankincense, lavender, marjoram, peppermint, rosemary (apply to temples, back of neck, and forehead)
Heart pounding	Lavender, melissa, orange, peppermint, ylang-ylang
Increased appetite and weight gain	Lemon and grapefruit "drink": Add five drops of each essential oil in 1 gallon/4.5 liters of water and drink throughout the day. Fresh grapefruit juice and lemon juice can be used instead.
Insomnia	Angelica, clary sage, cypress, lavender, lemon, marjoram, myrtle, orange, ravensara, rosemary, sandalwood, ylang-ylang (bathe in any of these before bed or drop on pillow)
Joint and muscle pain	Birch, ginger, juniper, nutmeg, rosemary, spruce
Menopausal-like hot flashes	Bergamot, clary sage, fennel, peppermint (apply to the ankles)

Sources: Connie Higley, Alan Higley, and Pat Leatham, *Aromatherapy A–Z*; Alison Wood, "Common Scents," *Look Good Feel Better,* 21 in *Chatelaine* (August, 2001).

Evening Primrose Oil: An Essential Fatty Acid

Evening Primrose Oil is an essential fatty acid, which is why it's useful for certain premenstrual discomforts. Essential fatty acids give us energy, maintain body temperature, insulate our nerves, and cushion and protect body tissues. The two essential fatty acids we need are linoleic acid (LA) and alpha linoleic acid. Both of these come from "good fats" and form prostaglandins in our bodies, which can either increase or decrease inflammation. Prostaglandins lower our blood pressure, reduce the risk of clots, and strengthen our immune system. When we have a diet high in "bad fats" we make prostaglandins that tend to increase inflammation. When we eat a diet rich in "good fats" we convert LA into gamma-linoleic acid, which helps to make the kind of prostaglandins that decrease inflammation, reducing breast pain and tenderness and even headaches and depression. Ingesting Evening Primrose Oil helps to convert LA into gamma-linoleic acid.

Other health problems such as hypothyroidism (see Chapter 4, "The Physical Premenstrual Signs") can further block this conversion of LA into GLA, which will increase inflammatory prostaglandins.

Herbs and Spices That Improve Digestion and Bloating

Many women suffer from premenstrual abdominal bloating, gas, and constipation. In addition to increasing fiber in the diet (see Chapter 6), they should consider trying the following herbs and spices that can aid digestion premenstrually — or anytime!

- **Coriander.** Eases gas and works to tone the digestive system. Use powdered or whole seed, or use fresh leaves (cilantro) as a garnish.

- **Cardamom.** Reduces the mucus-forming effects of dairy products. Use powdered or whole seeds.

- **Turmeric.** Generally improves metabolism and helps you to digest proteins. Use the root ground. (Gives dishes a yellowish color and can stain clothes and china.)

- **Black pepper.** Stimulates appetite and helps you digest dairy products. Use freshly ground.

- **Cumin.** Helps reduce gases and generally tones the digestive system. Use seeds whole or powdered.

- **Fennel.** Helps prevent gas. Chew the seeds after eating or add them to vegetables that tend to produce gas, when cooking. Use whole or powdered.

- **Ginger.** Aids digestion and respiration. Also helps to relieve gas and constipation, or indigestion. Use root fresh or dried. (Note: ginger can aggravate bleeding ulcers, however.)

- **Cinnamon.** Naturally cleanses your digestive system. Use powdered or in sticks or pieces.

- **Nutmeg.** Helps your body absorb nutrients from food, but should be used sparingly.
- **Clove.** Helps your body absorb nutrients. Use whole or ground.
- **Cayenne.** Helps to stimulate your digestive juices and is known for having a "cleansing action" in the large intestine. Helps to relieve that feeling of "fullness" after eating a heavy meal.

Alfalfa, dandelion, chickweed, nettle, and uva ursi can also be used as remedies for bloating.

Homeopathy for PMS

Homeopathy began in the early 19th century as a reaction to the "heroic measures" commonly used to treat disease at that time, such as bloodletting, inducing vomiting, and applying massive doses of drugs. Samuel Hahnemann, a German physician trained in conventional medicine and chemistry, founded homeopathy because he was disillusioned with conventional approaches to disease.

Homeopathy is based on the theory that "like cures like," or what Hahnemann called the Law of Similars. Essentially, the theory is that a substance that produces certain symptoms in a healthy person can cure a sick person who shows the same symptoms. He coined the term *homeopathy* from the Greek *homoios* and *pathos* ("similar sickness").

To treat disease, a homeopath will use minute doses of substances instead of large amounts. Hahnemann found he could preserve the healing properties and eliminate the side effects of a medication through a pharmacological process he called "potentization," in which substances are diluted with distilled water. The more diluted a substance, the more potent it was found to be. As a result of this discovery, Hahnemann proposed the controversial Law of Infinitesimals, which basically states that good things come in small quantities. In fact, to prove the theory, Hahnemann constantly referred to the minute amounts of hormones our bodies produce, which are so potent they govern our bodies.

Homeopathy was particularly popular in the 19th century for treating infectious diseases — particularly epidemics. "Homeopathy is often confused with "holism," but they're actually different disciplines. Homeopaths call their approach holistic because they believe they're treating not just one organ, but the entire patient. They see symptoms as positive signs that the body is trying to defend itself against an underlying disease. In fact, homeopathic drugs might even aggravate symptoms. A homeopath will say that a worsening of symptoms is really a sign that the body is stimulating its own self-healing mechanism.

Homeopathy involves very long medical history-taking sessions. Homeopaths use more than 2,000 remedies, all derived from various plant, mineral, animal, and chemical sources. Some examples include marigold flowers, onions, graphite snake venom, honeybee extract, and other wild concoctions. These treatments may sound dangerous, but since the doses are so diluted, they are widely recognized as harmless at worst in the general population.

Specific Homeopathic Remedies

The following are homeopathic remedies for common PMS complaints. Bear in mind that personality and specific groups of complaints are key in homeopathy. One cure does not fit all, and remedies are highly individualized. This information is provided not for self-treatment but for self-education in consultation with a qualified homeopathic practitioner. In general, the following are used for complaints as described:

- **Bovista:** For bloat and water retention, especially in the presence of diarrhea.
- **Calcarea carbonica:** Helps remedy fatigue and anxiety in the presence of all the physical discomforts, such as bloat, weight gain, food cravings, tender breasts, etc., as well as too-frequent periods lasting a long time. Chills and clammy hands and feet may also be discomforts that indicate the use of this remedy. (Note: This group of problems may indicate a thyroid disorder, too.)
- **Caulophyllum:** Best for women with a history of irregular cycles and infertility. Used to help relieve joint pain.
- **Chamomilla:** This remedy is best for women who have all the premenstrual mood changes, such as anger and irritability, in the presence of hypersensitivity to pain.
- **Cimicifuga** (also called *Actaea racemosa*): This remedy can be helpful for women with a history of irregular and painful periods who suffer from premenstrual back pain, headaches, muscle aches and pains, as well as premenstrual depression and agitation.
- **Kreosotum:** This remedy can be helpful for women with a history of heavy flows and poor libido, who suffer from premenstrual headaches, nausea, and irritability.
- **Lachesis:** This remedy is helpful for women with a strong, intense personality who suffer from premenstrual congestion, headaches, flushing, surges of heat, and irritability accompanied by feelings of suspicion or jealousy.
- **Lilium tigrinum:** This remedy may be helpful for women who suffer from premenstrual rage, creating a "walking on eggshells" environment for those around her.

- **Lycopodium:** This is helpful for women who experience premenstrual appetite increases with food cravings, as well as abdominal bloating and gas.
- **Natrum muriaticum:** This remedy is helpful for a woman with a reserved personality (reserved on the outside; deeply emotional on the inside) who suffers from premenstrual depression and sadness, as well as migraines, backache, and salt cravings.
- **Nux vomica:** This is a remedy for the woman who experiences premenstrual irritability in the presence of constipation.
- **Pulsatilla:** This remedy helps relieve general irritability, moodiness, and weepiness.
- **Sepia:** This is a remedy for a woman who suffers from premenstrual fatigue and lethargy.

Dosages

Usually the route homeopaths follow is to try one dose and wait for improvement. If there is no improvement, then taking the dose more frequently or at certain times may do the trick, or another remedy may be necessary.

Hands-on Healing for PMS

All ancient cultures, be they in native North America, India, China, Japan, or Greece, believed that there were two fundamental aspects to the human body. There was the actual physical shell (clinically called the corporeal body), that makes cells, blood, tissue, and so on, and there was an energy flow that made the physical body come alive. This was known as the life force or life energy. In fact, it was so central to the view of human function that each non-Western culture has a word for "life force." In China, it is called *qi* (pronounced chee). In India it's called *prana*; in Japan it's called *ki*, while the ancient Greeks called it *pneuma*, which has become a medical prefix having to do with breath and lungs.

Today, Western medicine concentrates on the corporeal body and does not recognize that we have a life force. However, in non-Western and ancient healing, it is thought that the life force that heals the corporeal body, not the other way around!

Just like the life force, every non-Western healer looks upon the parts of the body as "windows" or "maps" to the body's health. In China, the ears are a complex map, with each point on the ear representing a different organ and part of the psyche. In reflexology (discussed in Chapter 5, "Finding a PMS Doctor") it is the feet or hands that are "read" to tell us much about the rest of the body and spirit. In Ayurveda the tongue is read, while other traditions read the iris of the eyes, and so on. Western medicine doesn't really do this. Instead it looks at every individual part for symptoms of a disease and treats each part individually.

One of the most ancient forms of healing involves energy healing, which can involve therapeutic touch or healing touch. Technically, these techniques are considered forms of biofield therapy. An energy healer will use his or hands to help guide your life force energy. The hands may rest on the body or just close to the body, not actually touching it. Energy healing is used to reduce pain and inflammation, improve sleep patterns and appetite, and reduce stress. Energy healing, supported by the American Holistic Nurses Association, has been incorporated into conventional nursing techniques with good results. Typically, the healer will move loosely cupped hands in a symmetric fashion on your body, sensing cold, heat, or vibration. The healer's hands are then placed over areas where the life force energy is unbalanced in order to restore and regulate the energy flow. There may be clear benefits for hands-on healing in PMS.

Therapies that help to move or stimulate the life force energy include:

- Healing touch
- Huna
- Qi Gong

- Reiki
- SHEN therapy
- Therapeutic touch

All forms of hands-on healing work in some way with the life force energy.

Massage

Also discussed in Chapter 5, massage is more technically referred to as soft-tissue manipulation. Some benefits of massage include improved circulation, improved lymphatic system, faster recovery from musculoskeletal injuries, soothed aches and pains, reduced edema (water retention), and reduced anxiety.

Types of massage include

- Deep-tissue massage
- Manual lymph drainage
- Neuromuscular massage

- Sports massage
- Swedish massage

You can also massage pressure points yourself to relieve PMS discomforts. Here are some ideas.

To Calm Your Nervous System.

With the thumb of one hand, slowly work your way across the palm of the other hand from the base of the baby finger to the base of the index finger. Then rub the center of your palm with your thumb. Push on this point. Repeat this using the other hand.

To Relieve a Headache.

Grasp the flesh at the base of one thumb with the opposite index finger and thumb. Squeeze gently and massage the tissue in a circular motion. Then pinch each fingertip. Switch to the other hand.

For General Stress Relief.

Find sore pressure points on your feet and ankles. Gently press your thumb into them and work each sore point. The tender areas are signs of stress in particular parts of your body. By working them, you're relieving the stress and tension in various the organs, glands, and tissues. You can also apply pressure with bunched and extended fingers, the knuckles, the heel of the hand, or a gripping motion. Use this technique for self-massage on the hands, too, looking for tender points on the palms and wrists. Also use this technique to self-massage the ears. Feel for tender spots on the flesh of the ears and work them with vigorous massage. Within about four minutes the ears will get very hot.

Osteopathic Manipulation

Osteopathy is about the relationship between your body structure and your body function. If you correct anatomic structure by working your joints and muscles so that they "fall" correctly, like the shoulders on a dress or jacket, then you can restore health and wellness. Osteopathy involves manipulating your body parts in a variety of ways.

Osteopathic manipulation is a hands-on healing technique used by an osteopathic practitioner. It involves many of the same kinds of hands-on diagnostic approaches used by a family doctor (pressing various points to gauge whether there's pain, difficulty breathing, etc.). But it also involves much more attention to things like your posture and gait (the way you walk), overall flexibility and mobility, straightness of the spine, and so on. An osteopath will carefully examine your skin, too, looking fluid retention, muscular changes, temperature variations, and tenderness. The osteopath will then use hands-on healing techniques to manipulate and stimulate muscles, circulation, and so on. This may be combined with standard medical treatment in certain cases, but osteopathic manipulation tends to work well to relieve the physical symptoms of stress. One of the most common forms of osteopathic manipulation is "postural drainage," which is a technique used to mechanically unplug fluid blocks in the body to promote blood circulation.

"Postural Re-education" Strategies

Another popular form of hands-on healing is using touch to guide your body into better posture and alignment, similar in some ways to chiropractic healing. "Postural re-education," as it is called, involves using touch. By learning better posture, coordination, and balance, you relieve structural and functional stress. Three of the most common postural re-education methods used in North America are the Alexander technique, the Feldenkrais method, and Trager psychophysical integration.

The Alexander technique involves the repositioning of the head, neck, and shoulders. Developed by Australian actor Frederick Matthias Alexander (1869–1955), it involves being verbally guided into better posture and alignment through exercises that may involve lying, sitting, standing, or walking. At the same time, you'll be helped with areas that have posture-related tension. By avoiding certain movements, you can greatly decrease back pain or back problems, improve overall health, and improve your mental health with better focus, more patience, and so on.

The Feldenkrais method was developed by physicist Moshe Feldenkrais. He believed that movement, thought, speech, and feelings are a reflection of self-image, and argued that people made aware of their habits related to motion can be taught to move more easily and gracefully, resulting in improved self-image and better health. A combination of verbal guidance and gentle touch are used to make you aware of customary movement patterns and possible alternatives. More graceful and aware movements can improve stress-related symptoms and overall health.

The Trager method was developed by Milton Trager, M.D. (1908–1997) and is often called the Trager approach. This involves learning the joy of movement. Healers practicing this method use their hands to direct you through exercises involving bouncing, rocking, shaking, compression, and elongation. It is believed that using and moving your body in all ways it can be moved improves mindset, flexibility, and overall health, and reduces stress-related tension. Trager was born with a spinal deformity and through this method developed an athletic and graceful body.

8

NATURAL
PROGESTERONE
THERAPY FOR PMS

C hances are, you probably found some answers for even your more severe premenstrual discomforts in the previous chapters. If all else fails, natural progesterone therapy is the next thing to try. This therapy is widely prescribed for a range of women's health problems, especially for relieving menopausal discomforts (see Table 8.1 to understand why progesterone is so important to women's health).

The first doctor to promote the use of natural progesterone as a specific therapy for premenstrual discomforts (or what the medical community defines as PMS or PMDD) was Dr. Katharina Dalton, whom I introduced to you in Chapter 1. Dalton and others, such as Dr. John Lee (known more widely than Dalton), absolutely swear by natural progesterone therapy and insist it is a cure-all for many reproductive problems. These days, most physicians are open to natural progesterone therapy as a remedy for PMS, and many will prescribe it over synthetic hormones or oral contraceptives. But the studies comparing the efficacy of natural progesterone as a therapy for PMS remain sketchy; this has a lot to do with problems surrounding who "qualifies" as having "true PMS." There are also problems with the wrong lab tests being used to diagnose progesterone deficiencies, too. See the section titled "The Trouble with Natural Progesterone Studies" later in this chapter.

TABLE 8.1   What Progesterone Is Normally Supposed to Do in the Body

Major Actions of Progesterone

Maintains the uterine lining with secretions

Counterbalances breast stimulation

Helps convert fat into energy

Acts as natural diuretic

Acts as natural antidepressant

Facilitates thyroid hormone (counterbalanced by estrogen)

Normalizes blood sugar levels (counterbalanced by estrogen)

Normalizes blood clotting

Increases libido

Normalizes zinc and copper levels

Restores cell oxygen levels

Stimulates bone-building cells

Note: When it's balanced with estrogen, progesterone helps protect against many diseases, such as breast cancer or uterine cancer.

Source: A. Rushton and Dr. Shirley Bond, *Natural Progesterone*, 4.

Dalton's "Progesterone Receptor" Theory

Dalton's pioneering work led her to discover that PMS is not so much a problem of progesterone deficiency, but one that involves the functioning of the progesterone receptors. Progesterone receptors are like the taxis that transport progesterone to the body's various progesterone receptor sites (the taxi stands), which are located in the areas that control emotions in the brain; the eyes; the nasal passages; breasts; lungs; liver; and uterus, to name a few. So when the receptors are not working, not enough progesterone gets to the body's cells.

Progesterone receptors don't work in the presence of the following:

- **Adrenaline.** We pump out adrenaline while under stress and when our blood sugar is low. See Chapter 4 for details.
- **Low blood sugar levels.** This can occur from a high-carbohydrate, low-fat diet, when we are not spacing our meals properly. It can also occur when we suffer from eating disorders, or when we have too much insulin. See Chapters 4 and 6 for details.

What about Progestin?

Progestin is the synthetic version of progesterone that is found in all combination oral contraceptives; the injectable contraceptive, Depo-Provera; and the transdermal form, Norplant. Progesterone receptors do not recognize progestin and will not transport it to the cells. This may account for many of the progestin-related side effects that mimic PMS, discussed in Chapter 9, "Prescription Drugs Used for PMS." The most common progestins include Provera, Amen, Curretab, and Cycrin (all brand names of medroxyprogesterone acetate); Duralutin, Gesterol LA, Hylutin, Hyprogest (all brand names of hydroxyprogesterone caproate); Norlutate, Norgestrel, Aygestin (all brand names for norethindrone acetate); Norlutin (norethindrone); and Magace (megestrol acetate). Micronor, Nor-Q.D., and Ovrette are other brand-name progestins on the market.

Fixing the Progesterone Receptors

Eliminating the things that block the progesterone receptors can make them work, without the need for natural progesterone therapy. A proper diet that stabilizes blood sugar is one route. Trying to manage stress is another route, but it's not always effective. Going off progestins is a third route, if that's possible. When these approaches fail, taking natural progesterone, starting with high doses, will apparently kick-start the receptors again, fix the problem, and ease PMS.

John Lee's "Estrogen Dominance" Theory

Dr. John Lee is the next big name in the natural progesterone story. In the mid-1990s he published his theory that many women are progesterone-deficient due to estrogen dominance. Table 8.2 shows the role estrogen normally plays in the body.

Estrogen dominance can be caused by synthetic estrogens in oral contraceptives or other hormone therapies; obesity, because fat cells make estrogen; estrogen pollution caused by the flushed "pee" of women on all these synthetic estrogens getting into our sewage systems and water supply; another form of pollution known as environmental estrogens, also called xenoestrogens, which are beyond our control; and hormones in meat. Estrogen dominance can cause myriad health problems for women. Table 8.3 shows the signs of estrogen dominance. Unless there is an equal ratio of progesterone to estrogen, estrogen dominance can mean a progesterone deficiency. And for some women, that translates into severe PMS.

TABLE 8.2   What Estrogen Is Normally Supposed to Do in the Body

Major Actions of Estrogen

Decreases libido

Impairs blood sugar control (counterbalanced by progesterone)

Increases blood clotting (counterbalanced by progesterone)

Increases body fat (counterbalanced by progesterone)

Interferes with thyroid hormone (which is counterbalanced by progesterone)

Reduces oxygen levels in cells (counterbalanced by progesterone)

Reduces vascular tone

Retains salt and fluids

Slows bone loss (counterbalanced by progesterone)

Stimulates breasts (counterbalanced by progesterone)

Thickens the lining of the uterus (counterbalanced by progesterone)

Note: When estrogen is not counterbalanced by progesterone, many of these normal functions can turn into diseases, such as breast cancer or uterine cancer.

Source: A. Rushton and Dr. Shirley Bond, *Natural Progesterone*, 4.

TABLE 8.3 Signs of Estrogen Dominance

Accelerated aging	Headaches
Allergies (asthma, rashes, sinus congestion)	Hypoglycemia
Autoimmune disorders	Hypothyroidism
Blood clots and risk of stroke	Infertility
Breast tenderness	Insomnia
Cervical dysplasia	Irregular cycles
Decreased libido	Irritability
Depression, anxiety, and agitation	Memory loss
Difficulty concentrating	Miscarriage
Dry eyes	Mood swings
Early menstruation	Osteoporosis prior to menopause
Fatigue	PMS
Fibrocystic breasts	Slow metabolism
Fibroids	Uterine cancer
Gallbladder disease	Water retention/bloating
Hair loss	Weight gain

Source: Anna Rushton and Dr. Shirley Bond, *Natural Progesterone*, 6.

What Are Environmental Estrogens?

Environmental scientists have begun to notice that several wildlife species are experiencing hermaphroditic traits. In one area of the Florida swamplands, alligators are simply not breeding. A concerned research team from the University of Florida went into the swamps to find out why. These researchers pulled male alligators out of the water to examine their genitals. The majority of male alligators they found were sterile as a result of either non-developed or abnormally shaped penises. A chemical spill in nearby waters was found to be the culprit, which was having an "estrogenic effect" on the alligators' natural habitat.

Meanwhile, 1,500 miles north, in a Canadian creek near Lake Superior, scientists found that fish living close to a pulp mill in waters that contained certain chemicals with estrogenic effects, were now complete hermaphrodites. The male fish in these waters had developed ovaries and were sterile; the female fish had exaggerated ovaries. In other contaminated waters, fish had actually exploded from thyroid hormone overactivity.

Researchers in Sweden and the United Kingdom have been concerned since the late

1980s by a dramatic increase in male infertility in their countries, while there is an increased incidence of male infants being born with cryptorchidism, a condition in which the testicles do not descend into the scrotum but remain inside the abdomen. One study found that there has indeed been a huge decrease over the last 50 years in the quality of human semen. (A recent study measuring sperm quality in New York City contradicted these findings.) As well, the incidence of testicular and prostate cancers has greatly increased. In Britain, testicular cancer incidence has tripled over the last 50 years; it is now the most common cancer in young men under 30. In Denmark, testicular cancer has increased by 400 percent. As for prostate cancer, its incidence has doubled over the last decade. These male reproductive problems have been linked to environmental estrogens, too.

The scientific literature is slowly becoming saturated with findings linking one organic chemical after another to reproductive cancers and "endocrine disruption" in both wildlife and humans. Every study, from all corners of the world, is reaching the same conclusion: Organic chemicals are transforming into environmental estrogens. And they're everywhere. Organic chemicals are in the air we breathe from numerous air pollutants, in the food preservatives used in numerous canned and packaged goods, and in the pesticides used on fresh produce. These chemicals then contaminate the water and soil, which contaminate the entire human food chain.

Some suggest that environmental estrogens are "feminizing" the planet. Some suggest that women are being overloaded with estrogen, which may be associated with the rise of estrogen-dependent cancers, such as ovarian and breast cancer, as well as estrogen-related conditions, such as endometriosis (an estrogenic condition in which pieces of the uterine lining grow outside the uterus and can block the fallopian tubes) and fibroids. Estrogen pollutants are also thought to accumulate in fatty tissues (meaning they are stored in fat). Since women generally carry more body fat than men, women may be accumulating more of these toxins. Some studies have found that women with breast cancer tended to have higher concentrations of the organochlorines DDT, DDE, or PCBs in their fat tissue. In fact, elevated levels of DDE in the blood have been directly linked to a fourfold increase of breast cancer in the United States. We already know that dioxins, also organochlorines, are associated with endometriosis.

Some suggest that the environmental estrogen picture is equally dismal for men, many of whom are not only becoming slowly sterilized by this phenomenon, but are also developing reproductive cancers, as discussed above. Several prominent scientists have gone on record to say that this problem is *the* environmental priority of the 21st century!

On the flip side, many doctors point out that in the Western world, there has also been a huge increase in the "fatness" of the population. Obesity also increases the level of estrogen produced by our bodies.

Limiting Your Exposure to Environmental Estrogens

Right now, the only hope we have of eliminating environmental toxins is through consumer lobbying. The best place to start the environmental cleanup is in your kitchen. Your weekly groceries probably contain residues from pesticides and other organochlorines (on store-bought fruits and vegetables) and hormones in meat products, as well as a number of "extras" you may not have bargained for, which were fed to your meat when it was still alive. These include feed additives, antibiotics, and tranquilizers. Meanwhile, anything packaged will most likely contain dyes and flavors made from a variety of chemical concoctions.

Airborne contaminants, waste, and spills affect the water and soil, in turn affecting everything we ingest. When one species becomes unable to reproduce, we could lose not just that species but all those that depend on it, thus disrupting the food chain. Cleaning up the food chain is all part of creating a healthy, contaminant-free diet for ourselves. So check out the following to make your grocery list for your next shopping trip:

- At **www.cfia-acia.agr.ca**, you can find out what your produce has eaten and whether it was injected with anything, what waters your fish has swum in, and what sprays were used on your produce.

- You can find "safe food" that is organically grown or raised through a number of natural produce supermarkets or get in touch with the Organic Trade Association (serving both Canada and the United States) at **www.ota.com.**

- You can find out more about your supermarket's produce buying habits by contacting the company's head office.

Since the word "consumer" comes from the word "consume" — to eat — becoming vigilant about our groceries is the only way to help change the food industry. Customers can have an incredibly powerful impact on any company. In the 1980s, it was the "vigilant consumer" who helped to make manufacturers more green friendly and value-conscious. In many instances, the sheer volume of complaints and letters from customers has completely changed not only certain companies' habits and policies, but also an entire industry. If enough customers boycott products and protest manufacturing or agricultural practices, the companies will change. Start lobbying for change, and bring new meaning to the adage "The customer is always right!"

The Trouble with Progesterone Studies

Eight double-blind trials comparing the effectiveness of a placebo to progesterone failed to produce good results. Critics of progesterone say there isn't solid science behind using natural progesterone as a therapy, while there is for tranquilizers and antidepressants. The problem is that most progesterone studies are flawed for any of the following reasons:

- The studies measure levels of progesterone hormone in the blood, instead of checking levels through the saliva, which is a more reliable way of checking progesterone levels — especially when dispensing progesterone in cream form.

- They are placebo-controlled trials. See Chapter 7, "An Herbal and Hands-on Approach," for more on this type of study. We find similar problems with herbal studies.

- There is no good test to check the functioning of progesterone *receptors*, where the problem lies, according to Dalton.

- People are working with inaccurate definitions of "true PMS."

- Women with severe, debilitating PMS are excluded from these trials for ethical reasons (it's not ethical to give someone who is suffering a placebo when a good "standard" therapy exists — like antidepressants!) So women with milder symptoms may get better from the placebo effect (see Chapter 7).

- There is a high dropout rate.

- Studies take a long time (six months) of daily recording, and participants may not always record their bodily changes accurately.

- The participants cannot be on any form of contraception, must be menstruating regularly, must not be planning a pregnancy for at least six months, and must not be taking any other medication.

- Other factors such as diet, stress, and smoking are not ruled out or considered in these trials.

Given all that, it's difficult to get clear results. PMS comprises over 150 different kinds of symptoms, too.

Where to Find Natural Progesterone

Natural progesterone therapy is not available everywhere. You can't just walk into a health food store and buy natural progesterone. You need a prescription from a doctor (although the doctor need not be an M.D.; some naturopathic doctors prescribe them, too). A doctor's prescription for natural progesterone has to be prepared from "scratch," requiring what is known as a compounding pharmacist. Not all pharmacies are compounding pharmacies, so ask your doctor or current pharmacist about where to go to get a prescription prepared. You can also call the International Academy of Compounding Pharmacists (IACP) or the Professional Compounding Centers of America, Inc. (PCCA) for the nearest compounding pharmacist in your area. Several Canadian compounding pharmacists are members of either or both organizations. You can reach the IACP at 800-927-4227 or at **www.iacprx.org;** and the PCCA at 800-331-2498 or at **www.pccarx.com**.

What you can get over-the-counter in some health food stores and natural pharmacies are creams containing botanical progesterone, which is progesterone that comes from plants such as wild yam. This is not harmful, but it will not be as pure as the progesterone your doctor prescribes, which often comes from soy and wild yam, too, but is a very *pure* extraction. The term "natural progesterone" does not mean it is "human"; it means that it is not synthetic. Natural progesterone is recognized by our progesterone receptors as if it were progesterone we made in our bodies.

Creams

Progesterone works very well in cream form. There are a few kinds:

- Creams that contain only progesterone in a carrier such as aloe vera or vitamin E
- Creams with progesterone and other essential oils or herbs
- Creams that contain progesterone and phyoestrogens (plant estrogens)
- Creams that contain progesterone and three kind of natural estrogen

Creams that contain estrogen are not for PMS; they're for menopausal women who are using natural hormone therapy to relieve estrogen loss and other menopausal discomforts.

Natural progesterone can also be found in an oil form (taken under the tongue), tablets, capsules, vaginal suppositories, vaginal gel, and in an injectable form.

Dosage Recommendations

There is no one dosage recommendation for natural progesterone as a therapy for PMS. Dosages are individualized to match your particular needs, cycles, reproductive history, premenstrual discomforts, and so on. Dalton, for example, likes to start her

PMS patients on high doses of 400-mg suppositories twice a day, or lower doses by intramuscular injection. She maintains that the high doses "kick-start" the receptors. But you'll find all kinds of approaches to doses. You'll need to discuss your dosage with a doctor who is familiar with natural progesterone therapy. Many naturopaths are more knowledgeable about it than primary care doctors or gynecologists, but you'll have to shop around. One route is to consult a compounding pharmacist and ask for some names.

Progesterone therapy for PMS can't begin under the following conditions:

- You have your PMS throughout the cycle rather than experiencing it before you menstruate and not at all after you ovulate. (Use the charts in Chapters 3 and 4 to track your emotional and physical signs.) This may mean there is something else going on other than PMS, or in conjunction with it, so natural progesterone is not the answer.

- You are taking an oral contraceptive (although some doctors and pharmacists report that you can add natural progesterone in low doses beginning day eight of your cycle simply to combat progestin-related side effects).

- You are not getting enough sleep and are consuming too much alcohol

- Your blood sugar levels are not stabilized (see Chapter 6).

Using Progesterone as a Contraceptive

Don't blame me if you get pregnant, but Dalton recommends the following recipe as a contraceptive: Take a daily low dose of progesterone ranging from 100 to 200 mg. Use a progesterone suppository starting with day eight of your cycle. Then you increase to the "optimum" progesterone dosage (to be worked out with your doctor) at ovulation (and *you'll* have to know when you're ovulating). And then you continue daily progesterone until your period. Sounds a bit confusing to me, which is probably why it fails as a contraceptive in so many women. But if you're gifted with truly understanding your fertility cycle, it may work beautifully. If you want to try this method, combine it with a barrier method of contraception, such as a diaphragm, condoms, female condom, or cervical cap. It's wise to avoid IUDs (intrauterine devices), as they can complicate PMS and menstrual discomforts.

If your doctor says:

> "There is no proof whatsoever that natural progesterone therapy works for PMS."

You can say:

> Are you familiar with the work of Dr. Katharina Dalton and Dr. John Lee, who have both been using natural progesterone therapy for years with great success? I have some reading material for you here.

(Prior to saying this, get yourself a copy of each of their books. Get Dalton's *Once a Month* and do a search for Lee on **www.chapters.ca** or **www.amazon.com**; he's written a few books on this. Present these as evidence to your doctor.)

9

PRESCRIPTION DRUGS USED FOR PMS

When it comes to most drugs, we know very little about how they interact in women's bodies. That's because until 1993, women were excluded from clinical trials that tested drug potency, side effects, and interactions. But there's a reason for that exclusion. Women, the elderly, minorities, and other vulnerable populations had a long history of being *abused* in medical research — to such an extent that public outcry demanded stronger regulations to protect them.

In the mid-1970s, in response to the horrors of thalidomide and DES (diethylstilbestrol), legislation was passed to protect pregnant women and women of childbearing age. For example, U.S. Department of Health and Human Services regulations deliberately exclude pregnant women from research. Thalidomide (marketed in 1958), a "morning sickness" drug that was not properly tested prior to release, caused severe limb deformities in the developing fetus. DES was administered from the 1940s until the early 1970s as a "miscarriage prevention" drug; it was later revealed to cause a rare form of vaginal cancer in "DES daughters" as well as reproductive problems in DES sons.

But in spite of protective legislation, more DES-like disasters loom as widespread use of fertility drugs, which may cause ovarian cancer in women who do not conceive, echo the same concerns raised by DES activists. Tamoxifen, an anti-estrogen drug that can cause endometrial cancer, is being administered to healthy women considered at high risk of developing breast cancer; its use raises similar questions of abuse. Most disturbing, the off-label prescribing (meaning that the drug was prescribed for a condition the drug was never approved to treat) of fen/phen, the former anti-obesity drug therapy widely prescribed to women, was an example of just what happens when the public is not protected. Fen/phen caused heart failure, and there were deaths associated with its use.

Drugs used to treat mental health problems in women have a shady history, too. Millions of women are prescribed tranquilizers for social problems that have more to do with oppression than medical disorders. The good news is that far fewer women are prescribed tranquilizers for "social ailments" today than 10 years ago; the bad news is that for the *same* social ailments they are instead prescribed antidepressants, which can have damaging side effects.

This chapter discusses what you need to know about the drugs you're taking to relieve premenstrual physical discomforts as well as mood changes. The message of this chapter is *informed consent* (defined in Chapter 5, "Finding a PMS Doctor"). Make sure you know what you're taking and that you are fully informed about side effects of all drugs you're prescribed. What you need to know is that prescription medication is an option, not a requirement. Some women are not presented with choices when it comes to their health. My job is to see that you are. If you are currently taking prescription drugs for PMS and are responding well, please don't think I'm telling you to go off your drug. I'm simply telling you what you may *not* have known before you went on it.

Hormonal Therapy

If you require hormonal therapy for PMS, it's best to look into *natural progesterone therapy*, discussed in the previous chapter. If you're a sexually active woman who needs oral contraceptive protection (and there are many of us in this group!), the most widely prescribed drug to relieve PMS and cramps, and to regulate your cycle and flow, is an oral contraceptive. *In spite of this, oral contraceptives have not been adequately studied for treating PMS and are known to exacerbate premenstrual and mood changes.*

Some physicians who work with natural progesterone therapy maintain that you can combine natural progesterone with an oral contraceptive to help combat side effects of synthetic estrogens and progestin. Some also insist that, when used properly, natural progesterone can work as an oral contraceptive, but this is *heavily disputed*. If you want to use natural progesterone as a contraceptive, you must use a backup barrier method of birth control such as condoms or a diaphragm unless you don't mind being called "Mommy."

What You Need to Know about Oral Contraceptives

If you don't smoke and are healthy, you can be on a combination oral contraceptive (OC) from the time of your first period (called menarche) right up until menopause. That's because there are a number of fringe health benefits to being on an OC, known by clinicians as "noncontraceptive benefits." Because OCs prevent ovulation, they will also prevent diseases associated with the ovaries, such as ovarian cancer, ovarian cysts, and endometrial cancer. In fact, if you have no children or have no plans to get pregnant and breast-feed, staying on an OC will have the same therapeutic effects on your ovaries as pregnancy and breast-feeding because it will "give your ovaries a break." The following are considered clear, undisputed benefits of OCs:

- They reduce the incidence of endometrial cancer and ovarian cancer.
- They reduce the likelihood of developing fibrocystic breasts, which may or may not be associated with breast cancer.

- They reduce the likelihood of developing ovarian cysts.

- OC users have less menstrual blood loss and have more regular cycles, which reduce the chance of developing iron-deficiency anemia.

- The severity of cramps and premenstrual discomforts are reduced.

- You'll see an improvement in what's called "androgen-related side effects," such as acne or unwanted facial hair (Table 9.2 later in the chapter includes list of androgenic side effects). Androgen is to the male body what estrogen is to the female body; it is the sex hormone that makes his body "go." But progestin, which is synthetic progesterone, can cause this kind of side effect.

- Some brands may improve your cholesterol levels.

At age 50, you can begin to go off your OC at annual or biannual intervals to see if you're in menopause.

Will I Get a Blood Clot?

If you're healthy and don't smoke, serious cardiovascular problems linked to OCs are rare in women placed on *low-dose* Pills. Nevertheless, it's important to make sure that you're not *already* at risk for blood clots. If you have a history of thrombophlebitis, pulmonary emboli, and other cardiovascular diseases, you should not be encouraged to take OCs. Your risk of blood clots also increases if you

- Smoke

- Don't exercise

- Are overweight

- Are over 50

- Are hypertensive or diabetic

- Have high cholesterol

Breast Cancer Risk

Okay — here's the deal: If you're under 35 and do not have a family or personal history of breast cancer, and if you are not considered at risk for breast cancer due to any other significant factor, oral contraceptives will most likely not increase your risk of breast cancer. That's because the combination Pills used these days are very low-dose Pills. Studies from the 1970s and early 1980s may not apply to women today because they studied the effects of much higher-dose Pills than the ones women take now.

That said, the official warnings in your Pill packets tell you that if you have a mother or sister with a history of breast cancer, a Pill containing estrogen can put you at greater risk for developing breast cancer prior to menopause. The warnings will also tell you that if you've been on oral contraceptives longer than eight years and/or began them early, you are considered to be statistically more at risk for breast cancer. One U.S. study found that women under 35 who used an estrogen-containing Pill for more than 10 years increased their risk of breast cancer by about 70 percent compared to women who never took oral contraceptives at all. There are also studies that showed no difference in breast cancer risk between women who had been on the Pill for 10 years compared to non-Pill users, as well as studies that showed a decreased risk in Pill users after the age of 45 (which is potentially very good news). Since less than 2 percent of all breast cancers are diagnosed in women under 35 anyway, the study showing an increased risk really shouldn't rattle you all that much because, in the final analysis, you're looking at a very small number. Instead of one in 500 women developing breast cancer before 35, that statistic increases to one in 300.

At any rate, if you're concerned about breast cancer and oral contraceptives, you may want to ask your doctor about the progestin-only Pill (POP), which is also called the "mini-Pill." For the record, women are more at risk for blood clots on oral contraceptives than they are for breast cancer, and the risk of unwanted pregnancy under the age of 20 should also be weighed.

Age, of course, is also a factor. Since breast cancer incidence increases with age, using oral contraceptives when you're over 35 can also increase your risk. But, just like hormone replacement therapy, we don't know whether the increase is only age-related or whether oral contraceptives truly contribute to the increase. Either way, you'll still get protection from ovarian and endometrial cancer.

For the record, a recent study showed no increased incidence in breast cancer in women who were taking an OC for 10 years or more no matter what their family histories, ethnicity, age, or place of birth. In fact, if oral contraceptives were truly linked to breast cancers, experts say that we would have seen a very distinct and dramatic rise in breast cancer by now in OC users. And we haven't.

Estrogen versus Progestin Side Effects

Synthetic hormones used in oral contraceptives — synthetic estrogen and progestin (the synthetic version of progesterone) — are often not well synthesized by our bodies, which can lead to a state of progesterone deficiency. This is why natural progesterone therapy is so popular now. When we are deprived of our natural progesterone, and have too much estrogen, we can experience low blood sugar and severe premenstrual discomforts and mood changes. In fact, progestin is believed to be the culprit behind severe premenstrual discomforts such as bloating and mood changes.

That said, many of the side effects you can experience on OCs are dose related. In other words, if you go on a lower-dose OC, your side effects may disappear. In some cases, you may even require a slightly higher-dose OC — particularly if you have a history of heavy uterine bleeding.

Tables 9.1 and 9.2 will help you sort out whether your side effects are caused by too high a dose of estrogen or too high a dose of progestin, the synthetic progesterone

TABLE 9.1   Estrogen-Related Side Effects

Caused by Too Much Estrogen	Caused by Too Little Estrogen
Bloating*	Bleeding/spotting days 1–9
Blood clots and related disorders	Continuous bleeding/spotting
Breast cysts	Flow decrease
Capillary fragility	Pelvic relaxation symptoms
Cervical changes	Vaginitis atrophic
Chronic nasal congestion	
Dizziness*	
Dysmenorrhea (painful periods)	
Edema (water retention)*	
Excessive vaginal discharge	
Flu symptoms	
Hay fever/allergies	
Headaches*	
Heavy flow and clotting	
Increase in breast size	
Irritability*	
Leg cramps*	
Nausea/vomiting*	
Spidery veins in the chest area	
Splotchy face	
Urinary tract infections	
Visual changes*	
Weight gain*	
Uterine enlargement	
Uterine fibroid growth	

* PMS-related

Source: R. P. Dickey, *Managing Contraceptive Pill Patients.*

that's in combination OCs. Too much progestin is what creates those "androgenic side effects," which are basically appearance-related (referred to sometimes as "nuisance side effects"): weight gain, acne, and facial hair. The older progestins can cause a complex chemical reaction in the body that basically makes more testosterone available, which is what causes these side effects. In fact, most women who discontinue their OC will do so because of the androgenic side effects (and that's understandable!). A low-dose *triphasic* OC with a low-activity selective progestin may help in some cases. If progestin-related side effects don't disappear, you may want to consider another form of birth control.

When your doctor prescribes an oral contraceptive for you, you should ask three questions:

1. What is the estrogen dose? (Anything above 30–35 micrograms is considered high.)

TABLE 9.2 Progestin-Related Side Effects

Caused by Too Much Progestin	Caused by Too Little Progestin
Acne**	Amenorrhea
Appetite increase*	Bleeding/spotting, days 10–21
Cervicitis	Bloating*
Depression*	Delayed withdrawal bleeding
Edema**	Dizzines*
Fatigue*	Dysmenorrhea
Flow length decrease	Edema*
Hirsutism**	Headache*
Hypertension	Heavy flow and clots
Hypoglycemia symptoms*	Irritability*
Jaundice**	Leg cramps*
Leg veins dilated	Nausea/vomiting*
Libido decrease*	Visual changes*
Libido increase**	Weight gain*
Oily skin and scalp**	
Rash and pruritis**	
Weight gain*	
Yeast infections	

* PMS related
** Caused by excess androgen

Source: R. P. Dickey, *Managing Contraceptive Pill Patients.*

2. Is the oral contraceptive monophasic or triphasic? (Triphasic OCs may not contain a triphased progestin.) This has to do with how much hormone is distributed over the course of the cycle. In theory, triphasic OCs distribute more even amounts of hormones throughout the cycle.

3. Which progestin "recipe" is in the OC? (The newer progestins, such as norgestimate or desogestrel, are considered to be far gentler on your body in terms of side effects. Gestodene is a third new progestin that has not yet been approved in North America, but is expected to be very soon.)

There is also another wrinkle to the progestin story. The new ones are now "selective." What this means is that they are closer in appearance and behavior to natural progesterone, which, in theory, spells *fewer side effects*. This still needs to be borne out in studies, however.

The bottom line is that you should be able to walk out of your doctor's office with the lowest-dose OC possible to prevent pregnancy or, as I like to say: ALAP — as low as possible. Ask your doctor to show you all the OC samples and play a role in selecting the one you want.

Different People Need Different OCs

If you have tender breasts, heavy periods, and clots, request a low-estrogen, full-progestin oral contraceptive. This is the type of OC that will bring your cycles under control.

If you tend to have acne, oily skin, unwanted hair other than on underarms and legs, and if you suffer from PMS and mood swings, request a low-progestin OC (either triphasic or a new progestin).

If you're not getting your period while on your OC, this is a sign that you need a low-progestin or new-progestin OC.

If you have been unable to tolerate a combination OC, you may want to request an extremely low-dose OC, such as Minestrin (this delivers 20 micrograms of estrogen).

Although migraine sufferers are on the "stay away from OCs" list, it's important to note that the side effects vary. In fact, about 33 percent of women on an OC will notice an improvement in migraine headaches, 33 percent will notice no change at all, while another 33 percent will notice that their migraines get worse, which means that for them, the OC is not a good choice.

If you're diabetic, stay on top of your blood sugar levels. Oral contraceptives can alter your insulin requirements. That's because the progestins used in combination OCs can decrease glucose tolerance and increase insulin resistance. See Chapters 4 and 6 for more information.

And finally, if you have high blood pressure and do decide to go on an OC, have your blood pressure checked every three months during your first year on the OC.

Spotting and Bleeding

Spotting is when you notice a slight pink discharge between periods and need to use one pad or tampon per day. Spotting usually lasts only a few days and is nothing to worry about. All that's happening is that your body is adjusting to the hormone content of your OC. Your OC is still effective. If your spotting persists throughout the cycle, it's a sign that you may be on the wrong dose of progestin. Your doctor will simply prescribe another brand if this is the case.

Bleeding outside of your period while you're on an OC is called "breakthrough bleeding" (BTB) and is somewhat heavier than spotting, but just as normal. In this case, you may need to use more than a pad or tampon per day. You may experience it for a few days in the first three months of taking an OC at a certain point in your cycle. BTB disappears after about three months. Again, if it persists, talk to your doctor about possibly switching to another brand.

When in your cycle you're experiencing spotting or bleeding makes a difference. If your episodes occur at beginning of your cycle, you probably need more estrogen and less progestin; if the episodes occur at the end of your cycle, you need a stronger progestin.

If you have unprotected sex before or after you went on your OC, sudden episodes of breakthrough bleeding or spotting can be a sign that you have chlamydia. Get screened for this. Tetracyline will treat the problem.

Most doctors will probably tell you to wait three months on your OC to see whether the spotting or bleeding resolves on its own. Of course, missing Pills, vomiting, or diarrhea can be a factor, too. If the spotting or bleeding persists after three months, your doctor will probably switch you to another brand, and in some cases, may give you estrogen supplements.

Some doctors are in the habit of telling their patients to take "two pills a day until the bleeding stops." This is bad medicine and will put you more at risk for estrogen side effects! Switch doctors — *before* you switch OCs — if this is the advice.

If You're on Other Medications

Keep in mind that if you're on antiepileptic medications, such as phenobarbital and phenytoin (Dilantin), or the anti-TB drug rifampin, your OC will not be as effective and is probably not a good choice for you.

Antibiotics, such as ampicillin, tetracyclines, cephalosporins, chloramphenicol, erythromycin, isoniazid, and sulfonamides, can also make your OC less effective. Antifungals taken orally can also interfere with the OC's efficacy. The rule is to make sure you tell your doctor or pharmacist about any medication you're on before you fill — or refill — your OC prescription.

Gonadotropin-Releasing Hormone Analogs

Gonadotropin-releasing hormone (GnRH) is often used in fertility treatment, which is questionable, but it's certainly an extremely questionable drug to take for PMS. GnRH analogs are "copycat" gonadotropin-releasing hormone that block your pituitary gland from making follicle-stimulating hormone (FSH) and luteinizing hormone (LH; see Chapter 2). As a result, your entire natural hormonal axis shuts down, and your body goes into a kind of postmenopausal state — not a good idea. Say no to this. There's absolutely no indication to use GnRH analogs for PMS.

Drugs That Help Breast Tenderness

Some doctors prescribe bromocriptine (Parlodel) twice a day from day 10 of your cycle to the start of your bleed, to relieve tender breasts. Bromocriptine should be prescribed only in absolutely severe cases, because it is a form of prolactin, which can block estrogen in the body with many consequences. Ask about all the side effects.

Other Popular PMS Prescriptions

A few other prescription drugs are commonly prescribed to relieve various premenstrual signs. Be sure to ask about side effects, and how these may affect other drugs or herbs you're taking.

Diuretics: "Water Pills"

A diuretic helps you urinate excess water, but it also makes you "pee out" calcium, and is not a good PMS remedy at all. If you're going to use one, be sure it's a brand that preserves potassium for electrolyte balance. (Even then, you can suffer from potassium loss). There are many natural diuretics available over the counter. If you must take a diuretic, top up your calcium (see Chapter 6).

Drugs That Inhibit Prostaglandins

Past studies have shown that taking prescription drugs that inhibit body chemicals known as *prostaglandins* during the last 10 days of the cycle will help reduce PMS. Prostaglandins are substances manufactured by the endometrium that help uterine contractions during and after labor. Shortly before your period starts, the amount of prostaglandins produced sharply increases. In fact, menstrual cramps may be a result of the presence of too much of the specific prostaglandin that causes contractions. Anti-inflammatory drugs, such as naproxen sodium (Anaprox), mefenamic acid (Ponstan), or ibuprofen (Motrin), help alleviate cramps. The problem with anti-inflammatory drugs is that they can be hard on the stomach and create upper gastrointestinal problems, so avoid if possible.

Anti-Anxiety Agents

Anti-anxiety agents are called anxiolytics; popular types are alprazolam and buspirone hydrochloride. These drugs are often prescribed along with antidepressants and have many side effects. They can also be addictive. *Ask about side effects, please.*

Antidepressants for PMS

Antidepressants are widely prescribed for PMS, as discussed in the introduction and in Chapter 1. Two-thirds of all antidepressant prescriptions are prescribed for women, *but they work in only 60 percent of users.* Furthermore, many women are told that they have to stay on antidepressants for the rest of their lives to avoid relapsing into more severe depressions, but the truth is, you can be weaned off an antidepressant so long as you're aware of the "withdrawal effects." So if you're on this stuff and want to come off, have a frank discussion with your doctor about designing a withdrawal strategy. Do *not* just stop taking the drug on your own. You must be monitored during weaning.

How to Say No to Antidepressants

Prescribing antidepressants is so prevalent in our current medical system, I felt this section was as necessary for your protection as a self-defense course for a woman living in a crime-ridden city. It's important to note that many women instinctively recoil from taking antidepressants, but often will try them after feeling bounced around and ignored by doctor after doctor.

Here is an actual case history of a PMS patient who was prescribed tranquilizers throughout the 1980s and antidepressants in the 1990s for her PMS. The following is the patient's story in her own words, pulled from the transcripts of a recent medical conference:

I always had trouble around my periods. In fact, the more I look back, the more I understand them now. I was a really happy child. But when I started getting my period, I started to get very depressed at times. But then I'd be fine and happy again. When I was younger, I didn't really notice or associate it with a cyclical pattern. When I got older, I realized that I went through this cycle of only 1 good week of the month. I could tell like clockwork when I ovulated, because I would have a drastic mood change.

I would feel perfectly fine—I'd be happy, I'd feel energetic, I'd be going about my business. Then, all of a sudden someone might say something, and I'd take it totally wrong or it would irritate me. Then I'd snap and I would feel very irritable from that point on. The closer it got to my period actually starting, the worse I would get. Then the tears would come, and the depression, and the feeling like "I want to get out of here" — anxiety attacks. Just awful. To the point where in the last few years, it got so bad that I just started seeing one doctor after another to try to find out what I could do about it.

Most of the time, when I went to doctors and discussed it, they tried to insinuate that I was just suffering from depression. I did have depressive symptoms, but I knew that they were like clockwork and they disappeared right with my period. And the symptoms didn't really reappear until I ovulated or shortly thereafter. That was really stressful for me to keep hearing. And it was very painful. In fact, it still bothers me to talk about it, because it was hard. I would sit there and wonder, "What's wrong with me? Why aren't they listening to me?" I feel perfectly normal. I feel happy. I'm productive at work. I feel like a good mother. I don't feel like a depressed person 24 hours a day, day in and day out. But the symptoms come on just like a clock, at the middle of the month. Right after I got through the first few days of my period, it would start to lessen, and I'd be back to normal. Doctors would tend to ignore that, I think, and suggest all kinds of depression medications, which I don't really like to take. ("Clinical crossroads," 1999: 368–375)

When Your Doctor Says…

I don't have answers for everything, but the following scripts are enough to get the message across to your doctor that you're well-read and in charge of your health.

If your doctor says:

> I think the best route is for you to start on an antidepressant.

You can say:

> Doctor, it's a fact that antidepressants have harsh side effects. Many women report a flat mood (not able to feel passionate about anything), feeling dragged out and tired, as well as a low sex drive. Many women have great difficulty coming off these drugs. I feel a less invasive approach is to my benefit, and I would like you to help me investigate other health conditions that may be aggravating my PMS, and changes I can make to my diet and lifestyle. I am also interested in finding out about herbal and nutritional supplements that may help.

If your doctor counters with:

> I'm concerned that, if left untreated, your symptoms may tend to get more severe. And I'm worried that the longer your depression goes untreated, the more you'll suffer from repeated episodes of depression. We can try fluoxetine (Prozac) and if that doesn't work, we can try other SSRIs—sertraline or paroxetine.

You can say:

> It makes more sense to me to at least consider starting me on St. John's wort. In some European countries, the use of St. John's wort has increased to more than that of the standard SSRIs, such as Prozac [fluoxetine].

If your doctor counters with:

> St John's wort is a weak antidepressant and is not as effective as the standard antidepressants. It can also induce mania.

Most of you can say:

> But Doctor, that's in people who are suffering from severe, major depression, where they can't get out of bed for two weeks straight! That's not my problem. It's my understanding that for *mild to moderate* depression, which is what *I* suffer from premenstrually, St. John's wort works. I think it is in my best interests to at least try an herbal alternative that is very low in side effects than start on a powerful antidepressant that has a range of side effects clearly listed in the CPS [Compendium of Pharmaceuticals and Specialties] — side effects that can even aggravate my PMS. And as for St. John's wort and mania, it's clearly listed in the CPS that *all* SSRIs can induce mania to much more severe degrees.

How Antidepressants Work

First, a bit of brain chemistry: When your brain wants to send your body a message, a brain cell releases a substance called serotonin, which is a neurotransmitter (a chemical that helps to send signals through the brain) that rules our moods. Serotonin then locks onto a "receptor" on a neighboring brain cell, which relays the message to the next brain cell. Normally, the "transmitting" brain cell — the cell the serotonin locks onto — will reabsorb serotonin, making less of it available. The problem is that when you're depressed, less serotonin is initially released by a particular brain cell (the presynaptic cell), creating *really* low levels when "reabsorption time" comes around. Low levels of serotonin are associated with darker moods and depression.

If you think of a washing machine, serotonin is like the water that flows in at certain times and is flushed out at certain times. Normally, enough water flows in and out. But the brain chemistry in depression is akin to low water pressure. It's like setting your washing machine on "high" only to find that the water level doesn't go beyond "low." Opening up the lid of your machine midcycle will stop the machine and keep what little water you *have* in the machine, preventing it from flushing out into your laundry sink.

Prozac and Sarafem

Prozac and Sarafem (fluoxetine hydrochloride) *block* reabsorption, keeping more serotonin available to you, which brightens your mood. What makes Prozac and Sarafem so special is that they block *only* serotonin, and no other neurotransmitter, which is why they are called a *selective* serotonin reuptake inhibitors (SSRIs).

Prozac is touted as either a "wonder drug" or "happy pill" — depending on whom you talk to. Prozac, introduced in 1987, is to antidepressants what penicillin was to antibiotics: a breakthrough. It was the first antidepressant to be well tolerated by the majority of people taking it, and the first antidepressant that, in many cases, actually made a world of difference for the person taking it. As of 1994, 200,000 Canadians were taking Prozac, the majority of whom were women. In 1997, more than 7 million prescriptions for antidepressants (some Prozac, some Prozac-like) were filled by Canadian pharmacies, and by 2000, over 13 million antidepressant prescriptions were filled by Canadians — most of whom were women.

Predecessors of Prozac were not as selective and blocked a whole bunch of other neurotransmitters in the process, which could cause a wide range of side effects, such as tremors, blurred vision, gastrointestinal problems (constipation, nausea, etc.), weight gain, and sexual dysfunction. It's not that Prozac has no side effects, but they're much milder than the older generation of antidepressants, known as tricyclic antidepressants and monoamine oxidase inhibitors (MAOIs), both of which were discovered accidentally in the 1950s in the search for a tuberculosis cure. MAOIs destroy an enzyme called monoamine oxidase and break down neurotransmitters, thus leaving available more serotonin and norepinephrine, another neurotransmitter that affects mood.

Side effects of Prozac include nausea, nervousness, insomnia, and a decreased desire for sex, which, for most women, is a *huge* side effect!

Bad Press and Prozac

More than 20 million people have used Prozac to date, but the drug has had some bad press. Reports of Prozac users being driven into agitated states, violence, rage, suicide, and mania have surfaced, but considering all the users of Prozac, these negative effects are said to affect a small minority of users. But critics of Prozac insist that these side effects are more common than is generally reported about Prozac. However, it's difficult to determine whether these effects are strictly related to Prozac, or related to the disorders, depression, or mindset of the individuals taking Prozac.

A newer study indicates that 25 to 35 percent of the benefits a typical person on antidepressants gets is simply the placebo effect: the belief that the drug is making him or her feel better. Although this study has been criticized, it makes the allure of Prozac and Prozac-like drugs less appealing.

Side effects such as a decline in sexual drive or an inability to achieve orgasm can have serious consequences for women suffering from PMS or depression, whose self-esteem and feelings regarding body image are compromised at the best of times. Switching to another type of antidepressant may help, or adjusting your dosage. Better yet, discuss being weaned off the drug and looking into alternatives discussed throughout this book.

After Prozac

Other popular Prozac-like drugs, made by competing manufacturers, include Zoloft, Paxil, Luvox, and Effexor (which blocks both serotonin and another neurotransmitter, norepinephrine, known therefore as an SNRI). These newer SSRIs are even more finely tuned than Prozac, and are reported to have fewer side effects. See Table 9.3 for details on generic names, dosages, and major side effects.

The problem with SSRIs in particular is that you can build up a tolerance to the initial dosage, which means that the antidepressant benefits may subside. In this case,

TABLE 9.3   Meet Your Antidepressant

Monoamine Oxidase Inhibitors (MAOIs)

Common side effects: High or low blood pressure (this may cause dizziness); drowsiness, dry mouth, constipation. These drugs should not be used with over-the-counter cold and allergy medications, antidiabetic drugs, narcotic painkillers, tricyclic antidepressants (unless the person was already on the tricyclic when starting this drug), or any SSRI.

Generic Name	Brand Name
Phenelzine sulfate	Nardil
Tranylcypromine	Parnate

Tricyclic Antidepressants (TCAs)

Common side effects: Vary between sedation or agitation, depending on the brand. Other common side effects include weight gain, dry mouth, blurry vision, low blood pressure, and sexual dysfunction (decreased interest in sex, problems with erection, and lack of orgasm in both women and men). Tricyclics should not be taken with narcotic painkillers, MAOIs (unless you are already on the MAOI when you begin the trycyclic), and should only be combined with SSRIs with careful monitoring.

Generic Name	Brand Name
Desipramine	Norpramin
Imipramine	Tofranil
Amitriptyline	Elavil
Nortriptyline	Aventyl
Doxepin	Sinequan
Trimipramine	Surmontil
Clomipramine	Anafranil
Maprotiline	Ludiomil
Protriptyline	Triptil
Amoxapine	Asendin
Trazodone	Desyrel

Selective Serotonin Reuptake Inhibitors (SSRIs)

Common side effects: Sexual dysfunction such as the inability to achieve orgasm (Luvox excepted), nausea and other gastrointestinal discomfort, diarrhea, sleepiness or insomnia, short-term memory loss, tremors, restlessness, muscle spasms and twitches, involuntary movements of the face, limbs, and trunk.

Generic Name	Brand Name
Fluoxetine	Prozac, Sarafem
Sertraline	Zoloft
Paroxetine	Paxil
Fluvoxamine	Luvox

TABLE 9.3   Meet Your Antidepressant (continued)

Serotonin- Norepinephrine Reuptake Inhibitors   **(SNRIs)**

Common side effects: SSRI-like side-effects, including agitation, nausea, headache, and gastrointestinal problems. Can cause high blood pressure, too.

Generic Name	Brand Name
Venlafaxine	Effexor
Nefazodone	Serzone

Reversible Inhibitors of Monoamine Oxidase A (RIMAs)

Common side effects: Headaches, sleep disturbances, dizziness, tremors, increased agitation or anxiety, gastrointestinal problems, heart palpitations, low blood pressure, dry mouth. Not to be combined with other tricyclic antidepressants.

Generic Name	Brand Name
Moclobemide	Manerix

the dosages need to be increased. You'll start on the lowest effective dosage of your SSRI and then it will be increased gradually. In Pharmacyspeak, this is known as "start low, go slow." See further on about questions to ask about your drugs.

Antidepressants don't always work. Some brains are more resistant to antidepressants than others. Your doctor may start you on an SSRI and, if that doesn't work, switch you to another SSRI, and sometimes a third or fourth. If you're still not responding within three to five weeks, you may be offered an older antidepressant, such as a tricyclic antidepressant or an MAOI (refer to Table 9.3).

SSRIs and Hypomania

One serious problem with SSRIs, in particular, is their tendency to induce mild mania (also known as hypomania) in women who have never had any prior episodes of it. In short, taking an SSRI could put you at risk for a more serious problem, known as bipolar disorder or manic depression. This situation can be a medication nightmare, as you struggle to find balance. You may bounce from one therapy to another and struggle with severe depression in between states of hypomania. When more serotonin is available to you, you can get "high" on it, meaning that you exchange your depression for an even more difficult condition to treat. This is a risk all physicians should discuss with you prior to putting you on any antidepressant medication. If you have a personal or family history of bipolar disorders, stay away from antidepressant medication.

Some doctors believe that misdiagnosis may be more the culprit than antidepressants. You may have simply been misdiagnosed with depression instead of manic-depression. In this case, "normal" to you may have been your mild high. You then sought out help only when you were low, or depressed, and were diagnosed with unipolar depression. The magnification of the mania due to the antidepressants is simply revealing your true condition.

Regardless of what causes the mania, what *is* clear is that antidepressants can be truly disastrous for women with bipolar disorder, or manic depression. First, they can increase the frequency of depressive episodes, pushing you into a chronic depression instead of "episodic" depression. Second, these next bouts of depression may become resistant to treatment with antidepressants, and may be accompanied by other symptoms, such as irritability and anxiety. Add PMS on top of that, and you have a nightmare on your hands.

Other Antidepressants

The following is a list of other antidepressants, which may be prescribed for PMS.

- **Bupropion (Wellbutrin).** This has a low incidence of side effects affecting sexual function and has less chance of triggering hypomania.
- **Nefazadone (Serzone).** This may be a less effective antidepressant but does not affect your sexual drive or sleep patterns as dramatically.
- **Mirtazapine (Remeron).** Rather than blocking serotonin absorption, this drug triggers nerve cells to release more serotonin and norepinephrine, another neurotransmitter.

Combination Therapy

A number of people taking antidepressants are diagnosed with "treatment-resistant depression." This means that your depression is not responding to first-line drug treatments, such as SSRIs. In these cases, a combination of drugs may be used to treat your depression. It's important to be monitored closely when taking any antidepressant; it is especially important when the following drugs are added to your therapy:

- **Lithium.** As many as half of all treatment-resistant depressions respond well to lithium, which may be combined with other medication.
- **Tricyclic antidepressants.** In many cases, adding a tricyclic to an SSRI works well as a combination.

- **Psychostimulants.** These drugs may be added if you are diagnosed with attention-deficit hyperactivity disorder (ADHD), in which case treatment with stimulants in addition to an SSRI would clearly be indicated (stimulants are the treatment of choice for ADHD). But if you have a history of substance abuse, psychostimulants are not a good idea: they can become addictive.

- **Estrogen.** Estrogen replacement may be prescribed along with your antidepressant if you are past menopause. Because estrogen is, by itself, a weak antidepressant, in some women high doses of estrogen alone has been shown to treat depression.

What to Ask about Antidepressants

All of the drugs discussed in this chapter are powerful. And only a few of the drugs used to treat depression have been mentioned by name in this chapter. Without exception, all of the drugs currently being prescribed for depression have a long list of mostly unpleasant, and sometimes debilitating, side effects.

So the first question you must always ask before you take any drug prescribed is, What are the side effects? Many doctors have ethical problems with disclosing all potential side effects of the drugs they prescribe because you might "freak out" if you knew about all *potential* side effects. It's akin to an airline passenger reading about all the things that could go wrong with a plane before she flies. Do you *really* want to know? I can't answer that question for you; only you can. You know your "information threshold" better than I do. But in general, your doctor will disclose the *common* side effects. The drug's manufacturer will also have patient information available toll free or on an advertised website. If you insist on being told about rare and unlikely side effects, your doctor and pharmacist cannot legally withhold this information from you. If they do, and you're willing to risk unnecessary anxiety in exchange for probably *way* too much information about your drug, then you can always look up the drug in the *Compendium of Pharmaceuticals and Specialties* (CPS), available in your local library. (Chances are you won't understand most of what you read because it's so technical, but if you take a photocopy to your doctor or pharmacist, he or she can explain what it says and probably alleviate some fears.)

For the record, most psychiatrists are in the practice of withholding anything but the most common and serious of side effects. They believe that full disclosure could actually put certain patients at risk for increased anxiety or a worsening of the symptoms the drugs are meant to alleviate. This is certainly a valid point, but you have the right to be fully informed if you want to be.

It's also crucial to ask how diet, certain activities, and exercise can affect your medications.

A Dozen More Questions

1. **What are the alternative therapies?** The entire point of this book is to tell you about alternative therapies for PMS. So if this is the first chapter you're reading because you're already taking antidepressants for PMS, go back.

2. **How do these drugs affect my fertility, pregnancy, or breast-feeding?** If your drugs should not be taken during pregnancy or breast-feeding, ask for safe alternatives.

3. **What other therapies will be combined with this drug?** Anything from estrogen and thyroid hormone to anticonvulsants could be combined with your drug. Therefore, you may need to repeat questions about side effects, as well as any effect on fertility, for each drug added to your "main course" drug. Make sure you'll be talking to a therapist or counselor as well.

4. **How long does it take before I begin to feel better?** You should be charting your moods after you begin medication to help gauge your progress.

5. **What drugs or substances should not be combined with this drug?** Can you have wine? Cough medicine? Caffeine?

6. **How does this drug interact with other prescription drugs or over-the-counter medications I'm taking?** Whether you're taking oral contraceptives or drinking herbal tea, find out!

7. **How does my medical history affect the potency or toxicity of this drug?** Have you had any major surgeries? Do you have diabetes? Do you have a history of seizures? The tricyclics can affect heart rhythm, for example, which would be a problem if you have heart disease. All kinds of problems can turn up if you don't ask this question.

8. **How long does the drug stay in my system after I stop taking it?** For example, are you planning to get pregnant in three months and are worried it may take longer than that for the drug to leave your body?

9. **Can I stop the medication as soon as I feel better?** Great question. And usually you'll be told, "No, because you may experience a recurrence, or even worsening of your symptoms shortly after going off your medication." Psychiatrists maintain that this is part of a withdrawal effect and that you can, indeed, be weaned.

10. **How long do I have to take this drug?** Often the answer is "for the rest of your life," but again, you can be weaned off of antidepressants.

11. **How often do I have to take the drug and when is the best time?** Some drugs need to be taken three times a day, some once a day. Some drugs need to be taken at bedtime, some with meals. Make sure you have all this information. It could make a difference between good and bad side effects, potency, or how long the drug stays in your system.

12. **What if I miss a dose?** Sometimes the answer is to double up; other times you're told to skip it and carry on. The answer entirely depends on your medication, manufacturer, and dosage.

A Word about Dosages

This is brain chemistry. Every brain has different chemistry, and therefore requires different dosages. What works for Jane's brain may not work for Joan's! Therefore, as discussed earlier, the "start low, go slow" philosophy is always the rule. If Jane is on a higher dosage than Joan for the same diagnosis, it doesn't mean that Jane is in worse shape than Joan. It simply means that it takes more of the drug to work in Jane than in Joan. It's like alcohol. Some people take longer to get drunk than others, based on their tolerance for alcohol and their ability to metabolize it. And since many people eventually build up immunity to the starting dose, higher doses of the drug may be required in time. That doesn't mean you're getting worse; it just means you're getting *used* to the drug and you need more of it to derive its benefits.

The Importance of Being Monitored

You need to be closely monitored while taking antidepressants, and in particular, when you're weaned off of them. If being monitored is not discussed, this is a bad sign. In this case, raise the issue yourself. If you're told that being monitored isn't necessary, you should seek a second opinion.

Informed Consent and Medication

The term "informed consent" sounds nice, but most ethicists will agree that it is a misleading term with respect to the health care provider–patient relationship. Legal scholars and ethicists have noted that the term can be misunderstood by health care providers to mean the following:

- If you decline treatment, you're not informed.
- Information is provided solely to obtain your consent.
- Your refusing treatment does not have to be as informed as *consenting* to treatment.

Legally, if you are subjected to a treatment without your consent, it constitutes battery. If you are treated without *adequate* informed consent, it constitutes negligence. This applies to consenting to medication, drug trials, or any other form of therapy. For more about your rights, see Chapter 5, "Choosing a PMS Doctor."

Resources

Links from Sarahealth.com

For more information about disease prevention and wellness, visit me online at **www.sarahealth.com**, where you will find over 300 links — including the following — related to your good health and wellness.

Menstrual Disorders and Endometriosis

Chronic Illness Resource Site
Chronic illnesses, including fibromyalgia, chronic pain, etc.
www.angelfire.com/hi/HeidiHomePage

Inlet Medical Inc.
Information for women experiencing pain during intercourse, pain during menstruation, infertility, endometriosis, difficulty with tampons as a result of a retroverted or tipped uterus, etc.
www.inletmedical.org

Center for Endometriosis Care (CEC)
Facts on diagnosis, education, and treatment. Free newsletter.
www.centerforendo.com

The Institute for the Study and Treatment of Endometriosis
www.endometriosisinstitute.com

Endometriosis Association
Information and support.
www.endometriosisassn.org

The Cycles Page
Web-based application for tracking your menstrual cycle.
www.cyclespage.com

Menstrual Migraine Network
Information about hormone-induced headaches.
wbgray.tripod.com/index.html

General Gynecological Health

American Health Care Association
www.ahca.org

American Medical Women's Association (AMWA)
www.amwa-doc.org

GYN 101
Information on how to be an informed health care consumer. Especially for younger women.
www.gyn101.com

Healthy Way Sympatico Health
Comprehensive health site for Canadians, with extensive list of reviewed links.
www.sympatico.ca/Contents/health

Mayo Clinic
www.mayohealth.org/home?id=SP4.1.7

Melpomene Institute
Nonprofit research organization dedicated to women's health and physical activity. Good source of information on exercise and menstruation.
www.melpomene.org

National Women's Health Resource Center
www.healthywomen.org

Gladrags
Environmentally friendly menstrual products.
www.gladrags.com

Lunapads
Environmentally friendly menstrual products.
www.lunapads.com

Many Moons
Environmentally friendly menstrual products.
www.pacificcoast.net/~manymoons

Pandora Pads
Environmentally friendly menstrual products.
www.pandorapads.com

Salon.com
Sharp, engaging web magazine for women with lots of great health information and advice.
www.salon.com

Women's Health Information Center
www.ourbodiesourselves.org

Emotional Health

American Association of Marriage and Family Therapy
www.aamft.org

American Association of Suicidology
www.suicidology.org

American Counseling Association
www.counseling.org

American Psychiatric Association
www.psych.org

American Psychological Association
www.apa.org

Anxiety Disorders Association of America
www.adaa.org

Association of Gay and Lesbian Psychologists (AGLP)
www.aglp.org

AtHealth.com
Mental health links, chat, bulletin board, etc.
www.athealth.com

Canadian Mental Health Association
www.cmha.ca

CFS Days
For sufferers of chronic fatigue syndrome and fibromyalgia. Information about signs and symptoms, research, diagnosis, treatment, and medications. Discussion and support group.
www.geocities.com/cfsdays

Chronic Fatigue Syndrome at About.com
chronicfatigue.about.com

Depression Knowledge Center
Put together by the World Federation for Mental Health, this very comprehensive site offers FAQs, events listings, organizations list, archive, and discussion.
www.depressionnet.org

International Society for Mental Health Online
www.ismho.org

Internet Mental Health
Information on disorders and treatment, with online diagnostic services and psychopharmacology index.
www.mentalhealth.com

Mental Health at About.com
Updated daily. With articles, forums, chat, and a newsletter.
www.mentalhealth.about.com

Mental Health Center
Answers to many of the questions you're too scared to ask.
www.mentalhealthcenter.com

Mental Help
Award-winning guide to mental health, psychology, and psychiatry online.
www.mentalhelp.net

National Alliance for the Mentally Ill (NAMI)
www.nami.org

National Association of Social Workers (NASW)
www. naswdc.org

National Center for Post Traumatic Stress Disorder (PTSD)
www.dartmouth.edu/dms/ptsd

National Institute of Mental Health (NIMH)
www.nimh.nih.gov

National Mental Health Association
www.healthtouch.com

Obsessive Compulsive Foundation
www.ocfoundation.org

Online Dictionary of Mental Health
www.shef.ac.uk/~psysc/psychotherapy

Society for Light Treatment and Biological Rhythms
For seasonal affective disorder (SAD) sufferers.
www.sltbr.org

Walkers in Darkness
Information, a forum, and chat rooms for depressives and their loved ones.
www.walkers.org

General Health

American Health Care Association
www.ahca.org

American Medical Association
www.ama-assn.org

American Medical Association Medical Glossary
Help with terms that may be used in an informed consent document.
www.ama-assn.org/insight.genhlth/glossary/index.htm

Canadian Medical Association
www.cma.ca

Center for Medical Consumers and Health Care Information
www.medicalconsumers.org

Family Internet

Information on diseases, conditions, treatments, prognoses, etc. With a health and diet file.

www.familyinternet.com

Food and Drug Administration (FDA)

Regulations and information on drugs and other products.

www.fda.gov

Health Information Highway

Comprehensive health care resource with discussion groups.

www.stayhealthy.com

Healthy Way at Sympatico.ca

Good source of information organized by medical condition. Self-assessment resources, useful links and monthly magazine.

www.healthyway.sympatico.ca

Intelihealth

Home to Johns Hopkins health information, as well as the U.S. Pharmacopeia database.

www.intelihealth.com

Mediconsult.com

A–Z medical directory with drug information, fitness, nutrition, news briefs, online events, forums, and chat.

www.mediconsult.com

Merck Manual

One of the most popular manuals used by doctors worldwide. Detailed information about thousands of conditions.

www.merck.com

National Institutes of Health (NIH)

Dedicated to providing the public with the latest information about different health issues and ongoing scientific research/special reports.

www.nih.gov

Pharmaceutical Information Network (Pharm InfoNet)

Good resource for drug development information.

www.pharminfo.com

Online Pharmacies

www.drugstore.com

www.genrx.com

www.pharmweb.net

www.cponline.gsm.com (Clinical Pharmacology Online)

Drug Databases

RxList

Free, searchable database of more than 4,000 prescription and over-the-counter medications.

www.rxlist.com

PharmInfo

Drug data with links to articles

pharminfo/drugdb/dbmnv.html

Natural/Alternative Medications and Therapies

MotherNature.com

Information on what natural remedies do and how to take them.

www.mothernature.com

Homeopathy Home

www.homeopathyhome.com

EarthMed.com

World's largest website dedicated to natural and alternative, practitioners, products, and services.

www.earthmed.com

Finding a Doctor

Royal College of Physicians and Surgeons of Canada
rcpsc.medical.org

Conventional Resources

General Women's Health

The Canadian Women's Health Network
Suite 203, 419 Graham Avenue
Winnipeg, MB R3C 0M3
Telephone: (204) 942-5500
Fax: (204) 989-2355
Clearinghouse: 1-888-818-9172
E-mail: cwhn@cwhn.ca
Website: www.cwhn.ca

The Centre for Research in Women's Health
790 Bay Street, 7th Floor
Toronto, ON M5G 1N8
Telephone: (416) 351-3732
Fax: (416) 351-3746
E-mail: crwh.research@utoronto.ca
Websites: www.utoronto.ca/crwh and www.womenshealthmatters.ca

Depression

Canadian Mental Health Association
National office: 2160 Yonge Street, 3rd Floor
Toronto, ON M4S 2Z3
Telephone: (416) 484-7750
Fax: (416) 484-4617
E-mail: cmhanat@interlog.com

Canadian Psychiatric Association
237 Argyle Ave, Ste. 200
Ottawa, ON K2P 1B8
Telephone: (613) 234-2815

Centre for Addiction and Mental Health
33 Russell Street
Toronto, ON M5S 2S1
Telephone: (416) 595-6878
Fax: (416) 595-6881
Website: www.camh.net

Clarke Institute of Psychiatry
250 College Street
Toronto, ON M5T 1R8
Telephone: (416) 979-2221

Mood Disorders Associations Provincially (Listed West to East)

British Columbia

Mood Disorders Association of British Columbia
201-2730 Commercial Drive
Vancouver, BC V5N 5P4
Telephone: (604) 873-0103
Fax: (604) 873-3095

Alberta

Depression and Manic Depression Association of Alberta
Box 6404
Edmonton, AB T5K 2J5
Telephone: (888) 757-7077
Fax: (403) 987-4596

Organization for Bipolar Affective Disorders
1019 7th Avenue South West
Calgary, AB T2P 1A8
Telephone: (403) 263-7408

Saskatchewan

Society for Depression and Manic-Depression in Saskatchewan
2526 Comberland Ave. South
Saskatoon, SK STJ 2A2
Telephone: (306) 343-7518 (will provide further information on regional offices throughout Saskatchewan)

Manitoba

The Society for Depression and Manic Depression of Manitoba
4-1000 Notre Dame Avenue
Winnipeg, MB R3E ON3
Telephone: 1-800-263-1460, (204) 786-0987
Fax: (204) 783-4898

Ontario

The Mood Disorders Association of Ontario and Toronto
40 Orchard View Blvd., Suite 222
Toronto, ON M4R 1B9
Telephone: (416) 486-8046
Fax: (416) 486-8127

Mental Health Program Service
121 Kennedy Avenue, Suite 100
Toronto, ON M6S 2X8
Telephone: (416) 763-2188
Fax: (416) 763-2199

Quebec

Association des Depressifs et des Maniaco-depressifs
801 Rue Sherbrooke Est, Bureau 300
Montreal, PQ H2L 1X7
Telehpone: (514) 529-7552
Helpline: (514) 529-5619
Fax: (514) 529-9877

Nova Scotia

Depressive and Manic Depressive Society of Nova Scotia
c/o 73 Howe Street
Sydney, NS B14 4T9
Telephone: (902) 539-7179

Hotlines

Depression Information Resource & Education Centre (DIRECT)
1-888-557-5051, ext. 8000.
Also visit the DIRECT website:
www.fhs.mcmaster.ca/direct
1-800-THERAPIST
(1-800-843-7274.)
This is a referral resource.

Diabetes/Hypoglycemia

Canadian Diabetes Association

National Office
15 Toronto St., Suite 800
Toronto, ON M5C 2E3
Telephone: (416) 363-3373
Fax: (416) 363-3393

British Columbia/Yukon Division
1091 West 8th Ave.
Vancouver, BC V6H 2V3
Telephone: (604) 732-1331; 1-800-665-6526
Fax: (604) 732-8444

Alberta/NWT Division
Suite 1010, Royal Bank Building
10117 Jasper Ave. N.W.
Edmonton, AB T5J 1W8
Telephone: (403) 423-1232
1-800-563-0032
Fax (403) 423-3322

Saskatchewan Division
104-2301 Avenue C.N.
Saskatoon, SK S7L 5Z5
Telephone: (306) 933-4446; 1-800-996-4446
Fax: (306) 244-2012

Manitoba Division
102-310 Broadway
Winnipeg, MB R3C 0S6
Telephone: (204) 925-3800/1-800-782-0175
Fax: (204) 949-0266

Association Diabète Québec
(Quebec CDA affiliate)
5635 Sherbrooke Ave. East
Montreal, PQ H1N 1A2
Telephone: (514) 259-3422
Fax: (514) 259-9286

New Brunswick Division
165 Regent St., Suite 3
Fredericton, NB E3B 7B4
Telephone: (506) 452-9009; 1-800-884-4232
Fax: (506) 455-4728

Nova Scotia Division
6080 Young St., Suite 101
Halifax, NS B3K 5L2
Telephone: (902) 453-4232
Fax: (902) 453-4440

Prince Edward Island Division
P.O. Box 133
Charlottetown, PE C1A 7K2
Telephone: (902) 894-3005
Fax: (902) 368-1928

Newfoundland/Labrador Division
354 Water St., Suite 217
St. John's, NF A1C 1C4
Telephone: (709) 754-0953
Fax: (709) 754-0734

Food/Nutrition

The Canadian Dietetic Association
480 University Ave., Suite 601
Toronto, ON M5G 1V2
Telephone: (416) 596-0857
Fax: (416) 596-0603

Dietitians of Canada
To find a dietician in your area go to
www.dietitians.ca

National Institute of Nutrition
302-265 Carling Ave.
Ottawa, ON K1S 2E1
Telephone: (613) 235-3355
Fax: (613) 235-7032

Bibliography

Alcohol and Diabetes — Do They Mix? Booklet. Canadian Diabetes Association, 1996.

Allardice, Pamela. *Essential Oils: The Fragrant Art of Aromatherapy.* Vancouver: Raincoast Books, 1999.

Allen, Paula Gunn. *Grandmothers of the Light: A Medicine Woman's Sourcebook.* Boston: Beacon Press, 1991.

American Diabetes Association. "Carbohydrate Counting: A New Way to Plan Meals." Posted to *Diabetes.com*, January 1999.

Angier, Natalie. "In a Culture of Hysterectomies, Many Question Their Necessity." *New York Times*, February 17, 1997.

——. *Woman: An Intimate Geography.* New York: Houghton Mifflin, 1999.

"Antidepressants' impact mainly from boost of getting treated, study suggests." Associated Press, July 20, 1998.

Apple, Rima D., ed. *Women, Health and Medicine in America: A Historical Handbook.* Rutgers University Press,1992.

Arch Fam Med. 8 (March/April 1999): 122–128.

Baker Miller, J. "The development of women's sense of self." In *Women's growth in connection,* edited by J.V. Jordan, et al. New York: The Guilford Press, 1991, 11–27.

Baker, Sandy. "The Number One Way to Eliminate Daily Stress." *National Public Account* 144, no. 10 (December 2000): 13.

Ballweg, Rachel. "7 Simple Ways to Reduce Stress." *Better Homes and Gardens,* January 2000, 62.

Barnard, N.D , A. R. Sciallo, D. Hurlock, and P. Bertron. "Diet and sex-hormone binding globulin, dysmenorrhea, and premenstrual symptoms." *Obstet Gynecol.* 95 (2000): 245–250.

Bauer, Gabrielle. "You. Live and Undrugged." *Chatelaine,* July 2000.

Beck, Leslie. *Leslie Beck's Nutrition Guide for Women.* Toronto: Prentice Hall, 2000.

Bellafante, Ginia. "Who put the 'me' in feminism?" *Time,* June 29,1998.

Ben-Ari, Elia T. "Take Two Exercise Sessions and Call Me In the Morning." *BioScience* 50, no. 1 (January 2000): 96.

——. "Walking the tightrope between work and family." *BioScience* 50, no. 5 (May 2000): 472.

Bequaert Holmes, Helen. "A Call to Heal Medicine." In *Feminist Perspectives in Medical Ethics*, edited by Helen Bequaert Holmes and Laura M. Purdy. Indiana University Press: 1992.

Berndl, Leslie. "Understanding Fat." *Diabetes Dialogue* 42, no.1 (Spring 1995).

Beyers, Joanne, "How sweet it is!" *Diabetes Dialogue,* 42, no.1 (Spring 1995).

Bowen, Jon. "Fisticuffs in the cube: Stressed-out office workers are succumbing to 'desk rage.'" *Salon.com.* Sept. 7, 1999.

Breen, Mary J., "Poverty and Ill Health." *The Healthsharing Book: Resources for Canadian*

Women. Toronto: Women's Press, 1985, 150.

Breggin, Peter R. *Toxic Psychiatry.* New York: St. Martin's Press, 1991.

Breggin, Peter R., and Ginger Ross Breggin. *Talking Back to Prozac.* New York: St. Martin's Press, 1994.

Bullough, Vern L., and Bonnie Bullough. *Contraception: A Guide to Birth Control Methods.* Buffalo: Prometheus Books, 1990.

Burkman, Ronald T. *Handbook of Contraception and Abortion.* Boston: Little, Brown, 1989.

Burstow, Bonnie, "Women and Therapy." In *The Healthsharing Book: Resources for Canadian Women.* Toronto: Women's Press, 1985, 112.

Burstow, Bonnie, and Don Weitz. *Shrink Resistant: The Struggle against Psychiatry in Canada.* Vancouver: New Star Books, 1998.

Cain, Joanna M., and Albert R. Jonsen. "Specialists and Generalists in Obstetrics and Gynecology: Conflicts of Interest in Referral and an Ethical Alternative." *The Jacobs Institute of Women's Health* 2, no. 3 (Fall 1992).

"Calcium may be the key to taming premenstrual pain." Retrieved online from: www.cnn.com (August 25, 1998).

"Calcium supplements not equally effective." Reuters, Dec 27, 1999. *American Journal of Therapeutics* 6 (1999): 303–311, 313–321; and *Journal of Clinical Pharmacology* 39 (1999): 1–4.

Canadian Diabetes Association. "Physical Activity." *Equilibrium,* 1996.

Canadian Panel on Violence against Women. *Changing the Landscape.* Ottawa: Ministry of Supply and Services, 1993.

Caplan, Paula J. *They Say You're Crazy: How the World's Most Powerful Psychiatrists Decide Who's Normal* (New York: Addison-Wesley, 1995).

Casper, Robert F., and Alcide Chapdelaine. "Estrogen and Interrupted Progestin: A New Concept for Menopausal Hormone Replacement Therapy." *American Journal of Obstetrics and Gynecology* 168 (April 1993).

Cass, Hyla. *St. John's Wort: Nature's Blues Buster.* New York: Avery, 1998.

Chaddock, Brenda. "Activity is key to diabetes health." *Canadian Pharmacy Journal* (March 1997).

——. "Foul Weather Fitness: The hardest part is getting started." *Canadian Pharmacy Journal* (March 1996).

——. "The Magic of Exercise." *Canadian Pharmacy Journal* (September 1995).

Chesler, Phyllis. *Women and Madness.* New York: Avon Books, 1972.

Chez, Ronald A., and Franklin J. Apfel. "Women's Health Care: Rights and Responsibilities." *The Jacobs Institute of Women's Health* 2, no. 3 (Fall 1992).

Chilvers, Clair. "Oral contraceptives and cancer." *The Lancet* 344 (November 19, 1994): 1378.

Choi, Salmon P. "Symptom changes across the menstrual cycle in competitive sportswomen, exercisers, and sedentary women." *Br J Clin Psychol* 34 (1995): 447–460.

Christie, Aschwanden. "Relief for PMS." *WebMD Medical News* (May 22, 2000).

Christmas Derrick, Rachel. "Less Stress on the Job." *Essence,* March 2000, 44.

Chuong, C. James, Earl B. Dawson, and Edward R. Smith. "Vitamin E in Premenstrual Syndrome." *Nutrition Research Newsletter* 10 (January 1991).

"Clinical Crossroads: Conferences with Patients and Doctors." *JAMA* 281 (January 27, 1999): 368–373.

Clute, Eva. "Tamoxifen — Breast cancer preventive or human carcinogen: 1997 update." Paper presented at the World Conference on Breast Cancer, July13–17, 1997, Kingston, Ontario.

Colborn, Theo, John Peterson Myers, and Dianne Dumanoski. *Our Stolen Future.* New York: Dutton, 1996.

"Combat job stress: Does work make you sick?" Retrieved online from: www.convoke.com/markjr/cjstress.html (February 12, 1999).

"A Complex Question of Odds: Hormones Versus No Treatment," *HealthFacts* 18 (January 1993).

Coney, Sandra. *The Menopause Industry: How the Medical Establishment Exploits Women.* Hunter House, 1994.

Constipation: Causes. Booklet. 1996, Boston University Medical Center.

"Consumer Guide to Shepherd's Purse." *Mother Nature.com News.* Copyright 2001.

Costin, Carolyn. *The Eating Disorder Sourcebook.* Los Angeles: Lowell House, 1996; and Chicago: Contemporary Books.

"Counseling can be bad for your health." (Published online by Victoria MacDonald, London.) April 4, 1998.

Coutts, Jane. "Hysterectomies overused, study finds." *Globe and Mail,* February 26, 1998.

Cronier, Claire. "Sweetest Choices." *Diabetes Dialogue* 44, no. 1 (Spring 1997).

Cumming, David C., Ceinwen E. Cumming, and Dianne K. Dieren. "Menstrual Mythology and Sources of Information." *American Journal of Obstetrics and Gynecology* 164 (February 1991).

Dadd, Debra Lynn. *The Nontoxic Home and Office.* Los Angeles: Jeremy P. Tarcher, 1992.

Dalton, Katharina. *Once A Month: Understanding and Treating PMS.* 6th ed. Alameda, CA: Hunter House, 1999.

Datao, Robert. "The Law of Stress." The International Stress Management Association. Retrieved online from www.datodevelopment.com, June 2000.

Davis, D. L., H. L. Bradlow, M. Wolff, et al. "Medical hypothesis: Xenoestrogens as preventable causes of breast cancer." *Environ. Health Prospect* 101, no. 5 (1993): 372–377.

Davis, Martha, Elizabeth Robbins Eshelman, and Matthew McKay. *The Relaxation and Stress Reduction Workbook.* Oakland, CA: New Harbinger, 1995.

DeMarco, Carolyn. "Keys to the highway." *Wellness MD* 3, no. 6 (November/December 1993).

———. "Military research: Endometriosis and environmental toxins linked?" *Wellness MD* 4, no. 2 (March/April 1994): 23

———. *Take Charge of Your Body: A Woman's Guide to Health.* Winlaw, B.C.: The Last Laugh, 1990.

"Depression medicines can kill women's sex drive." *Vancouver Sun,* May 5, 1997.

Dickens, B.M. "The Doctrine of Informed Consent." In *Justice Beyond Orwell.* Edited by R. S. Abella and M. L. Rothman. Montreal: Yvon Blais, 1985, 243–63.

——. "Health Care Practitioners and HIV: Rights, Duties and Liabilities." In *HIV Law, Ethics and Human Rights – Text and Materials.* Edited by Jaysuriya. New Delhi:UNDP Regional Project on HIV and Development, 1995, 66–98.

"Differential Response to Antidepressants in Women with Premenstrual Syndrome/ Premenstrual Dysphoric Disorder: a Randomized Controlled Trial," *Archives of General Psychiatry.* Vol. 56, pp. 932–939, October 1999.

"Douching hazards compounded." *Globe and Mail,* August 30, 1997.

Dreher, Henry, and Alice D. Domar. *Healing Mind, Healthy Woman.* New York: Henry Holt, 1996.

El-Abyad, M. S., et al., "Preliminary screening of some Egyptian weeds for antimicrobial activity." *Microbios.* 62, no. 250 (1990): 47–57.

Emanuel, Ezekiel J., and Linda L. Emanuel. "Four models of the physician-patient relationship." *Journal of the American Medical Association* 267, no.16 (1992): 2221–2226.

Endometriosis Network of Toronto. *Intent: A Newsletter For Women With Endometriosis* 3 , no. 1 (Spring 1993).

Engel, June V. "Beyond Vitamins: Phytochemicals to help fight disease." *Health News* 14 (June 1996).

——. "Eating Fibre." *Diabetes Dialogue* 44, no.1 (Spring 1997).

Ensler, Eve. *The Vagina Monologues.* New York: Villard, 1998.

"EPO — Superfood for the 90s." *Holistic Health & Healing News* (www.hhnews.com) Retrieved online May 2001.

Epstein, Samuel S. "Pesticides pose a life-long threat." *New York Times,* August 29, 1994, 14 [Letter].

Etchells, E., et al. "Disclosure." *CMAJ* 155 (1996): 387–91.

——. "Voluntariness." *CMAJ* 155 (1996): 1083–6.

Etchells, E, Gilbert Sharpe, et al. "Consent." *Canadian Medical Association Journal* 155 (1996): 177–80.

"Evening Primrose Oil and PMS." *Nutrition Research Newsletter* 10 (February 1991).

"Exercise: Guidelines to a Healthier You." Patient information. Bayer Inc. Healthcare Division, distributed 1997.

Feminist Therapy Institute. "Feminist therapy code of ethics." *Ethical decision making in therapy: Feminist perspectives.* Edited by E. J. Rave and C. C. Larsen (1995): 38–41.

Ferraro, Cathleen. "New Uses Of Chemicals Linked To More Illness." (Published online Scripps-McClatchy Western, December 10, 1997.)

"A Field Guide To Stress: A Conversation with Kenneth R. Pelletier, Ph.D." Selfcare archives 12/15/97.

Findlay, Deborah, and Leslie Miller. "Medical Power and Women's Bodies." In *Women, Medicine and Health.* Edited by B. S. Bolaria and R. Bolaria. Halifax: Fernwood, 1994.

Fisher, Berenice. "Alice in the Human Services: A Feminist Analysis of Women in the Caring Professions." In *Circles of Care*. Edited by E. Able and N. Nelson. New York State University Press, 1990.

Flattum-Riemers, Jan. "Norplant: A New Contraceptive." *American Family Physician,* July 1991.

Food and Drug Administration. "Nutrient Claims Guide for Individual Foods." *Special Report, Focus On Food Labeling*. FDA Publication no. 95-2289.

———. Tampons and Asbestos, Dioxin, & Toxic Shock Syndrome, July 23, 1999. Retrieved June 2001 from: www.fda.gov/opacom/catalog/ots_tss.html and www.fda.gov/fdac/features/2000/200_tss.html.

Fransen, Jenny, and I. Jon Russell. *The Fibromyalgia Help Book*. Smith House Press, 1996.

Fugh-Berman, Adrienne. *Alternative Medicine: What Works*. Tucson, Arizona: Odonian Press, 1996.

Fukuda, et al. *Annals of Internal Medicine* 121 (December 15, 1994): 953–9.

"Get Herbal Relief." *Prevention,* July 1999, 128.

Gilligan, Carol. *In A Different Voice*. 2nd ed. Boston: Harvard University Press, 1993.

Gimenez, Martha E. "Feminism, Pronatalism and Motherhood." In *Mothering: Essays in Feminist Theory*. New Jersey: Bowman and Allenfeld, 1983.

Grahn, Judy. "From Sacred Blood to the Curse and Beyond." In *The Politics of Women's Spirituality: Essays on the Rise of Spiritual Power within the Feminist Movement*. Edited by Charlene Spretnak. Doubleday, 1982.

Greenberg, Brigitte. "Stress Hormone Linked To High-Fat Snacking In Women." The Associated Press, April 4, 1998.

Greenspan, Miriam. *A New Approach to Women and Therapy*. 2nd ed. Blue Ridge Summit, PA: Tab Books, 1993.

Greenwood, Sadja. *Menopause Naturally: Preparing for the Second Half of Life*. California: Volcano Press, 1992.

Grout, Pam. "Tune out Stress." *Ingram's,* April 1995, 78.

Guidelines for Conducting Assessments of Capacity. Office of the Public Guardian and Trustee, Ontario Ministry of the Attorney General (the Queen's Printer for Ontario, June 7, 1996).

Gunawant, Deepika, and Gopi Warrier. *Ayurveda: The Ancient Indian Healing Tradition*. Element, 1997.

Haas, Elson M. "Anti-Stress Nutritional Program." HealthWorld Online. Retrieved from www.healthy.net, June 2000.

Harrison, Pam. "Rethinking obesity." *Family Practice,* March 11, 1996.

Hatcher, Robert A., Felicia Guest, Felicia Stewart, Gary K. Stewart, James Trussell, Sylvia Cerel Bowen, Willard Cates. *Contraceptive Technology, 1990–1992*. 15th revised edition. Edited by Byron Breedlove, Beth Judy, and Nadine Martin. New York: Irvington, 1990.

Healing Voices: Feminist Approaches to Therapy with Women. San Francisco: Jossey-Bass, 1990.

Heimlic, Jane. *What Your Doctor Won't Tell You: The Complete Guide to the Latest in Alternative Medicine*. New York: HarperPerennial, 1990.

Helen J. Batchelder. "St. John's Wort Found to Relieve Premenstrual Symptoms." *MotherNature.com News.* 2001.

Hendler, Saul Sheldon. *The Doctors' Vitamin and Mineral Encyclopedia.* New York: Fireside Books, 1990.

Hendren, John. "Popular herbal remedy reportedly fails potency tests." Associated Press, August 31, 1998.

Herring, Jeff. "Bring back passion to your everyday life." Knight Ridder/Tribune News Service, February 21, 2000, K0535.

———. "Use these 10 tips to manage stress." Knight Ridder/Tribune News Service, January 31, 2000, K0817.

———. "You can manage stress with HALTS." Knight-Ridder/Tribune News Service, May 22, 2000, K1632.

Higley, Connie, Alan Higley, and Pat Leatham, *Aromatherapy A-Z.* California: Hay House, 1998.

Ho, Marian. "Learning Your ABCs, Part Two." *Diabetes Dialogue* 43, no. 3 (Fall 1996).

Hoffman, David L. "The Nervous System and Herbal Remedies." *HealthWorld Online.* Retrieved from www.healthy.net, June 2000.

"Homeopathic Remedies for Menstrual Problems — PMS and Menorrhagia." *The Natural Pharmacy.* Copyright © 2000 Healthnotes, Inc. (www.healthnotes.com).

Houppert, Karen. *The Curse, Confronting the Last Unmentionable Taboo: Menstruation.* New York: Farrar, Straus and Giroux, 1999.

Hufnagel, Vicki. *No More Hysterectomies.* New York: New American Library, 1989.

Hunter, J. E., and T. H. Applewhite. "Reassessment of Trans Fatty Acid Availability in the U.S. Diet." *American Journal of Clinical Nutrition* 54 (1991): 363–9.

Hurley, Jane, and Stephen Schmidt. "Going with the Grain." *Nutrition Action,* October 1994, 10–11.

"IFIC Review: Uses and Nutritional Impact of Fat Reduction Ingredients." Washington D.C.: International Food Information Council, October 1995.

Jatrina, M. Wyatt, et al. "Efficacy of Vitamin B-6 in the Treatment of Premenstrual Syndrome: Systematic Review." *BMJ* 318 (May 22, 1999): 1375–81.

Jill R. Lavella. "Herbal Therapy as a Supplement in Treating PMS." In *Where Motivation and Enrichment Meet.* Copyright September 1997.

Joffe, Russell, and Anthony Levitt. *Conquering Depression.* Hamilton: Empowering Press, 1998.

Johnson, Catherine. *When to Say Goodbye to Your Therapist.* New York: Simon & Schuster, 1988.

Johnson, Jeff. "Will Our Stolen Future Be Another Silent Spring?" *Environmental Science & Technology News* 30, no. 4 (1996): 168–70.

Johnson, Lois Joy. "You Look Divine: Stress Management Techniques." *Ladies Home Journal,* January 2000, 92.

Johnson, S. R., C. McChesney, and J. A. Bean. "Epidemiology of premenstrual symptoms in a nonclinical sample: prevalence, natural history, and help-seeking behavior." *J Reprod Med* 33 (1988): 340–6.

Kaptchuk, Ted, and Micheal Croucher. *The Healing Arts: A Journal Through the Faces of Medicine.* London: British Broadcasting Corporation, 1986.

Kennedy, Stephen. "Endometriosis," *The Lancet* 339 (June 20, 1992).

Keville, Kathy, and Peter Korn. *Herbs for Health and Healing*. Rodale, 1996.

Keyishian, Amy. "Calming Rituals for Rotten Days." *Cosmopolitan*, February 2000, 152.

Kirk, Jo-Anne. "Gender inequality and medical education." In Bolaria and Bolaria, *Women, Medicine and Health*, 1994.

Kishi, Misa. *Impact of pesticides on health in developing countries: Research, policy and actions*. Paper presented at the World Conference on Breast Cancer, July13-17, 1997, Kingston, Ontario.

Kotulak, Ronald. "Researchers: Lack of sleep may cause aging, stress, flab." *Chicago Tribune*, April 5, 1998.

Kra, Siegfried J. *What Every Woman Must Know About Heart Disease*. Warner Books, 1996.

Kramer, Peter D., *Listening to Prozac*. New York: Penguin, 1993.

Lad, Vasant. *Ayurveda: the Science of Self-Healing*. Twin Lakes, WI: Lotus Press, 1984.

Lark, Susan, M. *Chronic Fatigue and Tiredness*. Los Altos, CA: Westchester, 1993.

———. *The Menopause Self Help Book*. Berkeley, CA: Celestial Arts, 1990.

Leary, Warren E., "A look at douches' safety," *New York Times*, April 29, 1997.

LeBlanc, Gerald A. "Are Environmental Sentinels Signaling?" [Commentary.] *Environmental Health Perspectives* 103, no. 10 (October 1995).

Ledochowski, M., B. Sperner-Unterweger, and D. Fuchs. "Lactose malabsorption is associated with early signs of mental depression in females: a preliminary report." *Dig Dis Sci* 43 (November 1998): 2513–7.

Lee, John R. *What Your Doctor May Not Tell You About Menopause*. New York: Warner Books, 1996.

Leibenluft, Ellen. "Why are so many women depressed?" *Women's Health* 9, no. 2 (Summer 1998).

Leutwyler, Kristin, "Dying to be thin." *Women's Health* 9, no. 2 (Summer 1998).

Levine, R. J. *Ethics and Regulation of Clinical Research*. New Haven: Yale University Press, 1988.

"Limited Dose of B-6 Appears to Aid PMS." *Alternative Health News*, www.altmedicine.com. May 22, 1999.

Lindsay, Robert. "Prevention and Treatment of Osteoporosis." *The Lancet* 341 (March 27, 1993).

Linton, Marilyn. *Taking Charge by Taking Care*. Toronto: Macmillan Canada, 1996.

Lurie, Nicole, Jonathan Slater, and Paul McGovern. "Preventive care for women: Does the sex of the physician matter?" *New Engl. J. Med.* 329, no. 7 (August12, 1993): 478.

Mains, Rachel P. *The Technology of Orgasm: "Hysteria," The Vibrator, and Women's Sexual Satisfaction*. Baltimore: John Hopkins University Press, 1999.

"Major causes of ill health." *Rachel's Environment & Health Weekly* #584 (Published online by the Environmental Research Foundation), February 2, 1998.

Maleskey, Gale, and Charles B. Inlander. *Take This Book to the Gynecologist With You: A Consumer's Guide to Women's Health*. New York: Addison-Wesley, 1991.

Margolis, Dawn. "After a 20-year Delay, a New Birth Control Method Hits the Market: Contraceptive Injection." *American Health*, March 1993.

Martin, Raquel. *The Estrogen Alternative: Natural Hormone Therapy with Botanical Progesterone.* Rochester, Vermont: Healing Arts Press, 1997.

Mason, J. K., and R. A. McCall Smith. "Prenatal Screening and Wrongful Life." In *Law and Medical Ethics.* 3rd ed. London, UK: Butterworths, 1991.

Mastroianni, Anna C., Ruth Faden, and Daniel Federman, editors. *Women and Health Research: Ethical and Legal Issues of Including Women in Clinical Studies,* Volume 1. Washington, National Academy Press, 1994.

Mattila, Antti. "Life At The Crossroads: Depression — Philosophical Perspectives." Paper presented at The Fourth International Conference on Philosophical Practice, August 3–7, 1998, Bergisch Gladbach, Germany.

Maurer, Janet. *How To Talk To Your Doctor.* New York: Simon & Schuster, 1986.

McConnell, Kathleen, and Mariana Valverde. *The Healthsharing Book: Resources for Canadian Women.* Toronto: Women's Press, 1985.

"Menstrual product resources." Retrieved June, 2001 from S.P.O.T. at: http://critpath.org/~tracy/spot.html.

Montgomery, Ann. "Truth About Tampons Needs To Be Told." *Ottawa Citizen,* September 1, 1992.

Morrison, Judith H. *The Book of Ayurveda.* New York: Simon & Schuster, 1995.

Murray, Michael T. *Premenstrual Syndrome.* New York: Prima Publishing, 1997.

Nechas, Eileen, and Denise Foley. *Unequal Treatment: What You Don't Know About How Women Are Mistreated by the Medical Community.* New York: Simon & Schuster, 1994.

Nelson, Philip K. "Defining Chronic Fatigue Syndrome." *The Manasota Palmetto,* January 1995.

Nichols, Mark. "Questioning Prozac." *Maclean's,* May 23, 1994.

Nicole Martin, Brande. "Low-fat, Vegetarian Diet Reduces PMS Symptoms." *JAMA Electronic Media.* Retrieved online May 2001.

"Numerous roadblocks keeping botanicals across border." *Globe and Mail,* September 28, 1998.

"Nutrients in fruit and vegetables linked to bone health." *American Journal of Clinical Nutrition* 71 (2000): 142–51.

Ontario Task Force on the Primary Prevention of Cancer. Recommendations for the Primary Prevention of Cancer: Report of the Ontario Task Force on the Primary Prevention of Cancer. [Toronto]: March 1995. Presented to the Ontario Ministry of Health.

"Oral Contraceptives and Venous Thromboembolism." *American Journal of Nursing* 10, no. 9 (September 1986).

Orbach, Susie. *Fat Is a Feminist Issue.* New York: Berkley Books, 1990.

Osofsky, Howard J. "Efficacious Treatment of PMS: A Need For Further Research." *The Journal of the American Medical Association* 264 (July 18, 1990).

Osteoporosis Society of Canada. "Calcium." Fact Sheet Series Number 3, 1999.

Palferman, T. G. "That Estrogen Replacement for Osteoporosis Prevention

Should No Longer be a Bone of Contention." *Annals of the Rheumatic Diseases* 52 (January, 1993).

Patient Information. The National Digestive Diseases Information Clearinghouse, (NDDIC) a service of the National Institute of Diabetes and Digestive and Kidney Diseases, part of the National Institutes of Health, under the U.S. Public Health Service. 1996, National Digestive Diseases Information Clearinghouse, Licensed to Medical Strategies, Inc.

Pearson, Cynthia. "FDA Waffles on Premarin Decision." *Network News,* July/August, 1990.

Pepper-Smith, Robert, William R.C. Harvey, and M. Silberfeld. "Competency and Practical Judgment." *Theoretical Medicine* 17, no. 2 (June 1996).

Perry, Susan, and Katherine O'Hanlan. *Natural Menopause: The Complete Guide to a Woman's Most Misunderstood Passage.* New York: Addison-Wesley, 1992.

Pierpont, Margaret, and Diane Tegmeyer. *The Spa Life at Home.* Vancouver: Whitecap Books, 1997.

Pincus, Jane. Introduction to the 25th Anniversary Edition of *Our Bodies, Ourselves.* In *Our Bodies, Ourselves: For the New Century.* New York: Simon & Schuster, 1998.

"Placebo or pharmacological effect with antidepressant." The Associated Press [online], July 20, 1998.

"PMS, Cramps, Delayed Menstruation & Heavy Bleeding." *MotherNature.com News,* 2001.

"PMS: What Causes It, How Diet Can Help." *WebMD,* 1999

"Pocket Partner: A Guide to Healthy Food Choices." Booklet. Canadian Diabetes Association, 1997.

"Pocket Serving Sizer. Patient Information." Canadian Diabetes Association, 1997.

Poirier, Laurinda M., and Katharine M. Coburn. *Women & Diabetes:Life Planning for Health and Wellness.* New York: American Diabetes Association and Bantam Books, 1997.

Pope, Tara Parker. "Drug Firms Treat PMS As a Mental Disorder." *Wall Street Journal,* February 23, 2001.

"Position of The American Dietetic Association: Use of Nutritive and Nonnutritive Sweeteners." *Journal of The American Dietetic Association* 93 (1993): 816–22.

"Postmenopausal Osteoporosis and Preventative Measures." *American Family Physician* 45, no. 3 (March 1992).

"Postmenopausal Osteoporosis and Synthetic Calcitrol." *American Family Physician* 43, no. 3. (March 1990).

"Prozac: Help or Hype?" *Health for Women,* Spring/Summer 1998.

"Putting fun back into food." International Food Information Council, Washington D.C., 1997.

"Q&A about Fatty Acids and Dietary Fats." International Food Information Council, Washington D.C., 1997.

Raloff, J. A. "Plastics may shed chemical estrogens." *Science News* 144 (July 3, 1993): 12.

Rand, Michael. "The Mayo Clinic Weighs In on PMS Relief." *MotherNature.Com News,* May 26, 1999.

Reaney, Patricia. "Report probes chemical link to disappearing sperm." Reuter's News Service, London, July 25, 1995.

Reid, Robert L. "Understanding Premenstrual Syndrome." *Synphasic Education Series* pamphlet.

Reilly, P. R., et al. "Ethical issues in genetic research: disclosure and informed consent." *Nat Genet* (January 1, 1997): 16–20.

"The return of sunny spring isn't the cure for all cases of seasonal depression. Sometimes it's the cause." Published online by Deborah Franklin, *Health Magazine*, 1996.

Roberts, Francine M. *The Therapy Sourcebook*. Chicago: NTC/Contemporary Publishing, 1998.

Rodriguez-Trias, Helen. Preface to the 25th Anniversary Edition of *Our Bodies, Ourselves*. In *Our Bodies, Ourselves: For the New Century*. New York: Simon & Schuster, 1998.

Rosenberg, L., J. R. Palmer, R. S. Rao, et al. "Case-control study of oral contraceptive use and risk of breast cancer." *Am. J. Epidemiol* 143, no. 1 (January 1, 1996): 25–37.

Rosenthal, M. Sara, *50 Ways To Prevent Colon Cancer*. Chicago: Contemporary, 2001.

———. *50 Ways To Prevent and Manage Stress*. Chicago: Contemporary, 2001.

———. *The Gynecological Sourcebook*. 3rd ed. Chicago: Contemporary Books, 1999.

———. *Managing Your Diabetes For Women*. Toronto: CDG Books, 1999.

———. *Stopping Cancer at the Source*. Vancouver: SarahealthGuides, 2001.

———. *The Thyroid Sourcebook*. 4th ed. Chicago: Contemporary Books, 2000.

———. *Women and Sadness: A Sane Approach To Depression*. Toronto: CDG Books, 2000.

———. *Women of the '60s Turning 50*. Toronto: Prentice Hall Canada, 2000.

Rosser, Sue V. *Women's Health — Missing from U.S. Medicine*. Indiana University Press, 1994.

Roth, Loren H., Alan Meisel, and Charles W. Lidz. "Tests of Competency to Consent to Treatment." *The American Journal of Psychiatry* 134, no. 4 (1977).

Rubin, Rita. "Birth control failure: Americans — and their doctors — ignore some effective options." *U.S. News & World Report*, March 3, 1997, 66–8.

Rudd, Wm. Warren. *Advice From The Rudd Clinic: A Guide To Colorectal Health*. Toronto: Macmillan Canada, 1997.

Rushton Anna, and Shirley A. Bond. *Natural Progesterone*. London, UK: Thorsons, 1999.

Salvatore, Steve. Web-post to www.cnn.com (New York), August 25, 1998.

Segal, Marian. "Norplant: Birth Control at Arm's Reach." *FDA Consumer Magazine*, May 1991.

Seto, Carol. "Nutrition Labelling — U.S. style." *Diabetes Dialogue* 42, no.1 (Spring 1995).

"Sex Under Siege." Documentary. 1994, Canadian Broadcasting Corporation.

Shaw, Robert W. "Treatment of Endometriosis." *The Lancet* 340 (November 21, 1992).

Sherwin, Susan. "Feminist and Medical Ethics: Two Different Approaches to

Contextual Ethics." In *Feminist Perspectives in Medical Ethics*, edited by Helen Bequaert Holmes and Laura M. Purdy. Indiana University Press, 1992.

Sherwin, Susan. *Patient No Longer: Feminist Ethics and Health Care.* Philidelphia: Temple University Press, 1984.

Shore, Laurence S., Michael Gurevitz, and Mordechai Shemesh. Estrogen as an environmental pollutant. *Bulletin of Environmental Contamination and Toxicology* 51 (September 1993): 361–6.

Shuttle, Penelope, and Peter Redgrove. *The Wise Wound: Menstruation and Everywoman.* New York: Marion Boyars, 1999.

"Sorting Out the Facts About Fat." International Food Information Council, 1997.

Soto, Ana M., Kerrie L. Chung, and Carlos Sonnenschein. "The Pesticides Endosulfan, Toxaphene, and Dieldrin Have Estrogenic Effects on Human Estrogen-Sensitive Cells." *Environmental Health Perspectives* 102 (February 1994).

Soto, Ana M., Honorata Justicia, Jonathan W. Wray, and Carlos Sonnenschein. "*p*-Nonyl-Phenol: An estrogenic xenobiotic released from 'modified' polystyrene." *Environmental Health Perspectives* 92 (1991): 167–73.

Spake, Amanda. "Our Worst Fears About Pesticides And Plastics May Be Coming True — If Maverick Researcher Devra Lee Davis Is Right." 1995 *HEALTH magazine*, Document ID: MASO95C.

Steege, J. F., and J.A. Blumenthal. "The effects of aerobic exercise on premenstrual symptoms in middle-aged women: A preliminary study." *J Psychosom Res.* 37 (1993): 127–33.

Stehlin, Dori. "Depo-Provera: The Quarterly Contraceptive." *FDA Consumer Magazine,* March 1993.

Steinem, Gloria. Preface to the 25th Anniversary Edition of *Our Bodies, Ourselves.* In *Our Bodies, Ourselves: For the New Century.* New York: Simon & Schuster, 1998.

Steingraber, Sandra. *Living Downstream: An Ecologist Looks at Cancer and the Environment.* New York: Addison-Wesley, 1997.

Stevens, William K. "Pesticides may leave legacy of hormonal chaos." *New York Times,* August 23, 1994, C1.

Stevinson, Ernst E. "A pilot study of Hypericum perforatum for the treatment of premenstrual syndrome." *Br J Obstet Gynaecol.* 107 (2000): 870–6.

"Strategic Eating." *Wellspring Media* (www.wellmedia.com). Retrieved online May 2001.

"Stress Affects Your Health More Than You Think." Posted online to www.mediconsult.com, September 9, 1999.

"Stress May Intensify Cold Symptoms." Posted online to www.mediconsult.com. March 26, 1999.

"Study Further Links Smoking To Depression." Reuters News Service, February 10, 1998.

Sturdivant, Susan. *Therapy with Women: A Feminist Philosophy of Treatment.* New York: Springer, 1980.

Szarewski, Anne, and John Guillebaud. "Contraception: Current State of the Art." *BMJ* 302 (May 25, 1991).

Szasz, Thomas. *Cruel Compassion: Psychiatric Control of Society's Unwanted.* New York: Wiley, 1994.

———. *The Myth of Mental Illness: Foundations of a Theory of Personal Conduct.* New York: Harper & Row, 1974.

Tampon Safety and Research Act of 1999, HR 890 IH, 106th United States Congress, 1st Session, 5H. R. 890. Presented In The House Of Representatives March 1, 1999.

Thompson, Rachel. "Toxins & Tampons." *WEED* 2, no. 2 (Spring 1999).

Thys-Jacobs, S., P. Starkey, D. Bernstein, and J. Tian, for the Premenstrual Syndrome Study Group. "Calcium Carbonate and the Premenstrual Syndrome: Effects on Premenstrual and Menstrual Symptoms." *Am J Obstet Gynecol* 179 (1998): 444–52.

Tisserand, Maggie. *Aromatherapy for Women.* Rochester, Vermont: Healing Arts Press, 1996.

"Toxics that tamper with hormones." *Eagle's Eye* [World Wildlife Fund Canada newsletter], Summer 1995.

"Update on the Ontario Task Force on the Primary Prevention of Cancer." City of Toronto Public Health Department, May 16, 1996.

Veatch, R.M. "Abandoning Informed Consent." *HCR* 25, no. 2 (1995): 5–12.

Walter, Carolyn. "The Dilemma of the Female Physician in the Feminist Health Center." *Journal of the American Medical Women's Association* 43, no. 2 (1988): 45–50.

Warren, Virgina, L., "Feminist Directions in Medical Ethics." In *Feminist Perspectives in Medical Ethics,* edited by Helen Bequaert Holmes and Laura M. Purdy. Indiana University Press, 1992.

Weed, Susun S. *Menopausal Years: The Wise Woman Way — Alternative Approaches for Women 30–90.* Woodstock, NY: Ash Tree Publishing, 1992.

———. *Wise Woman Ways: Menopausal Years.* Woodstock, NY: Ash Tree Publishing, 1992.

Weintraub, Amy. "The Natural Prozac." *Health World Online.* Posted to www.healthy.net, 2000.

Westcott, Patsy. *Thyroid Problems: A Practical Guide to Symptoms and Treatment.* London, UK: Thorsons/HarperCollins, 1995.

"What Is Endometriosis?" Endometriosis Association, Education Support Research Pamphlet, Milwaukee, Wisconsin, 1992.

"What is Intensive Diabetes Management?" [Patient information.] Diabetes Clinical Research Unit of Mount Sinai Hospital Toronto, distributed 1997.

"What You Should Know About Sugars." International Food Information Council, May 1994.

Whiteford, Linda. "Political Economy, Gender and the Social Production of Health and Illness." In *Gender and Health,* edited by C. Sargent and C. Brettell. Toronto: Prentice Hall, 1996.

Williams, Linda S. "International Conference on Reproductive and Genetic Engineering and Women's Reproductive Health." *Resources for Feminist Research* 18, no. 3 (1989).

"Women Find Themselves Courted By Pharmaceutical Firms." The Associated Press, July 20, 1998.

Wonnemann, M., A. Singer, and W. E. Muller. "Inhibition of Synaptosomal Uptake of H-3-L-glutamiate and H-3-GABA by hyperforin, a Major Constitutent of St.John's Wort: The Role of Amiloride Sensitive Sodium Conductive Pathways." *Neuropsychopharmacology* 23, no. 2 (2000): 188–97.

Wood, Alison. "Common Scents." *Look Good Feel Better.* Canadian Cosmetic, Toiletry & Fragrance Association Foundation, 2001.

Woods, N. F., M. J. Lentz, E. S. Mitchell, M. Heitkemper, J. Shaver, and R. Henker. "Perceived Stress, Physiologic Stress Arousal, and Premenstrual Symptoms: Group Differences and Intra-individual Patterns." *Res Nurs Health* 21, no. 6 (1998): 511–23.

Worell, J., and P. Remer. "A Feminist View of Counseling and Therapy." In *Feminist Perspective in Therapy: An Empowerment Model for Women.* New York: Wiley, 1992.

Wright, Diana. "Make No Mistake: New Improved Birth Control Gets Cleaner and Easier." *Chatelaine,* July 1998, 115.

Wright, Jonathan V., and John Morgenthaler. *Natural Hormone Replacement.* Petaluma, CA: Smart Publications, 1997.

"You are what you eat." *Equilibrium* [Canadian Diabetes Association], 1996.

"You have diabetes ... Can you have that?" [Booklet.] Canadian Diabetes Association, 1995.

"Your blood sugar level ... what does it tell you?" [Patient information.] Eli Lilly of Canada, 1997.

Zand, Janet. "Herbal Programs for Stress." *HealthWorld Online.* Retrieved from www.healthy.net, June 2000.

Zellerbach, Merla. *The Allergy Sourcebook.* Los Angeles: Lowell House, 1995.

Zimmerman, Mary K. "The Women's Health Movement: A Critique of Medical Enterprise and the Position of Women." In *Analysing Gender,* edited by M. Farle and B. Hess. Toronto: Sage, 1987.

Index

autoimmune diseases, 80–81
Ayurveda, 102: compared with Chinese medicine, 103

B

bacteria, friendly, 31
bad cholesterol. *See* LDL cholesterol
bad fats, 168
bad stress, 66
beauty, standards of, 36, 40, 41–42, 43–44, 143 (*See also* body image anxiety; eating disorders)
behavioral counseling. *See* cognitive-behavioral therapy
beneficence, 113 (*See also* nonmaleficence)
beta-carotene, 137–138
binge-eating disorder. *See* compulsive eating disorders
bioethics, 110–115
biofeedback, 105
biofield therapy, 172
bioflavonoids, 139
biopsychiatry, 57–58
bipolar disorder, 35, 39, 203–204
birth control pill. *See* oral contraceptives
birthdays, cause of depression, 40
bladder, endometrial growth in, 22
bleached tampons, 28–29
bleaches, exposure to, 27
bleeding: breakthrough, 195; heavy, 18–20; and OCs, 195; withdrawal, 25
blighted ovum, 16
bloating, xi, 6–7, 71, 128: and fiber intake, 133–134; homeopathic remedies, 170, 171; and magnesium, 137; natural therapies, 165, 166, 168–169; result of eating disorders, 143, 144; and sodium intake, 129–130
blood clots, OC risk, 190
blood coagulation disorder, 19
blood glucose test, 83
blood sugar (blood glucose), 6, 63, 71–72: and carbohydrates, 118–120; and estrogen, 82; low. *See* hypoglycemia; and moods, 118, 122; and progesterone, 82, 118; stabilizing, 118–127; versus PMS, 6, 82–86, 118
blood sugar reading, normal, 84
"Blue Book" listings (Ontario), 49
body image anxieties, 36, 41, 142–143 (*See also* beauty, standards of; eating disorders)
boron, 139
Boston Women's Health Book Collective, 107–108
botanical progesterone, 183
brain, 14, 39, 103, 177, 200, 207
"brain foods," 127, 128
breast-feeding, x, 25, 76, 189
breast tenderness, xi, 7, 137, 165, 166: drugs that relieve, 196
breasts, fibrocystic, 189
breath therapy, 105
breathing exercises, 149–150
bromocriptine (Parlodel), 196
bulimia nervosa, 143
bupropion (Wellbutrin), 204
burnout, 64 (*See also* chronic fatigue syndrome)
B vitamins, 127–128
Byers, Dwight D., 106

C

caffeine, 73, 74, 128, 135
calcium, 21, 128, 135–137, 143, 196
calendar month, 15 (*See also* Gregorian calendar)
cancer(s): breast, 5, 29, 180, 188, 190–191; cervical, 29; colon, 133; and dioxin exposure, 28, 29; endometrial, 25, 188, 189, 191; estrogen-dependent, 22, 180; lung, 74; ovarian, 25, 29, 99, 180, 188, 189, 191; prostate, 180; reproductive, 180; testicular, 180; thyroid, 87; uterine, 18; vaginal, 188
Candida albicans, 81

capacity/competency, informed consent, 112

Caplan, Paula, 7

carbohydrates, 118–125

carotenes, 139

Carson, Rachel, 55

catecholamines, 63

Centers for Disease Control and Prevention (CDC), 30, 79

cervix, 13, 22: cervical mucus, 15; cervicitis, 98

Chesler, Phyllis, 8, 96

Chinese medicine, 103: herbal preparation warning, 107; and massage, 105

chiropractic, 103

chlamydia, 195

chromium, 139

chronic fatigue immune deficiency syndrome (CFIDS), 79

chronic fatigue syndrome (CFS), 75: causes, 80–81; fibromyalgia versus, 80; symptoms, 79–80; treatment, 81–82

chronic illness, cause of depression, 42

chronic self-induced vomiting, 144

circadian rhythm sleep disorders, 47

cleanliness issue, menstrual cycle, 3, 15, 30–32

client/therapist relationship, 52–54 (*See also* health care provider/patient relationship)

clinical ecology, 104

clinical psychologists, 50

clots, 19, 190

Coalition for the Medical Rights of Women (Calif.), 108

cognitive-behavioral therapy, 56–57, 82, 130

College of Social Work, 51, 52

combination oral contraceptives, 25, 177, 189, 192–193: androgenic side effects, 190, 193

combination therapy, and depression, 204

community-based programs, 44–45

community family services, therapist source, 48

community services listings, therapist source, 49

Compendium of Pharmaceuticals and Specialties (CPS), 205

complaints, standards of practice, 115

complementary healing systems, 101–107

complex carbohydrates, 118, 119

compounding pharmacist, 183, 184

compulsive eating disorders, 144–145

confidentiality, 112

connection, sense of, 42, 44–45; power of, 56; with other women, 110

constipation: and eating disorders, 143–144; herbs/spices to alleviate, 168–169; pre-menstrual, 133

consumer(s): medical services, 94, 115; psychiatric, 35, 96–97; vigilance, foods, 181

continuous struggle, cause depression, 36

contraception: barrier methods, 20, 184, 189; oral. *See* oral contraceptives

copper, 140

corporeal body, 171

corpus albicans, 15

corpus luteum, 14, 15

cortisol, 76, 96

counseling services, community-provided, 52

counselor, 51, 52

cramping, 12, 21, 99, 137: and anti-inflammatories, 197; herbs to relieve, 160–161

creativity, stress-reliever, 152–153

credentials, academic, 49–52, 101, 106

crime, 6, 45 (*See also* violence)

crisis lines, 49

crying, 35, 132

cryptorchidism, 180

cultural attitudes: to menstrual cycle, 13; to PMS, 2–4

The Curse (Houppert), 4, 5

"the curse" (term), 12

cyclamate, 125, 126

cysts, ovarian, 20, 24, 25, 99, 189, 190

D

Dalton, Katharina, 5–6, 7, 63, 83, 95, 118, 176, 177, 183–184, 185

Danazol, 99

dawn simulator, 47 (*See also* light therapy)

D&Cs (dilation & curettage), 99

deep-breathing exercises, 149–150

Defoe, Daniel, 96

degrees, academic, 49–52, 101, 106

Depo-Provera, 25, 177

depression: diagnosing, 39; and diet, 28, 122; iatrogenic, 9; and loss of pleasure. *See* anhedonia; major, 9, 46; medicalization of, 5; neurology of, 200; and PMS, x, 6, 7, 34, 35–48, 134; post-meal, 122; social causes for, 35, 36, 39–45; statistics, 35; symptoms, 37–39; treatment-resistant, 204; treatments for, 31, 32, 47, 156, 161–165 (*See also* antidepressants); versus PMS, 6, 35, 37, 39; and weight issues, 38–39 (*See also* bipolar disorder; seasonal affective disorder; situational depression; unipolar disorder)

DES (diethylstilbestrol), 188

de-selfing concept, 46

dextrose, 125, 128, 129

DHEA (dehydroespiandrosterone), 164

diabetes, and OCs, 194 (*See also* Type 1 diabetes; Type 2 diabetes)

Diagnostic and Statistical Manual of Mental Disorders, Fourth Edition (DSM-IV), 6, 7–8, 39

diapers, 26, 28

diet: Ayurvedic approach, 102; to stabilize blood sugar, 118–127; and CFS, 81; contaminant-free, 181; healthy, 119; and stress, 127–128

diet books, 121

diets, 121

dieting, 143

digestion, natural remedies, 168–169

dioxins, 22, 28, 29, 180

disaccharides (double sugars), 129

disclosure, informed consent element, 111–112

diuretics, 196

divorce, cause for depression, 42

doctors, approach to PMS, 94–101

Domar, Alice, 42

domestic violence, 40–41, 45

dopamine, 63

doshas, 102

douching, 31

downshifting, 81

Dr. Atkins' New Diet Revolution, 121

Dreher, Henry, 105

D-tagatose, 127

drug identification number (DIN), 156

due awareness, health care provider, 115

dysmenorrhea (painful periods), 12, 21–25

dysphagia, 144

E

eating disorders, 6, 17–18, 41–42, 43, 45, 142–147

eco-feminism, 55

Effexor, 201

Ehrenreich, Barbara, 8

electrolyte balance, 196

Eli Lilly, x–xi, 9

emotional cycle chart, 59–60

employee assistance programs, therapist source, 48

endocrine disruption, organic chemicals, 180

endocrinologists, 19, 99

endometrial: growths, 22, 23; particles, 15; tissue, 24

endometriosis, 20: causes, 21–22, 29, 180; defined, 21, 22; diagnostic approach, 24; stages, 24; symptoms, 22–24; treatment, 21, 24, 99 (*See also* adenomyosis)

Endometriosis Assn., 23
endometrium, 16, 23, 24, 197
endorphins, 72, 102, 118, 132, 148
energy drains, 76–78
energy healing, 172
English, Dierdre, 8
Ensler, Eve, 4
environmental estrogens, 21, 178, 179–181
environmental medicine, 104
Environmental Protection Agency, 28
environmental toxins, 80–81
environmental triggers, depression, 40–45
epinephrine, 63 (*See also* adrenaline)
Epstein-Barr virus, 78
essential fatty acids (EFAs), 139, 167–168
essential oils, 31–32, 165, 166
estrogen: and blood sugar, 82; and fat cells, 76, 180; and fertility drugs, 42; and obesity, 181; role of, 14, 16, 20, 75, 178; too little, 6, 14, 192; too much, 6, 191–192 (*See also* cancers, estrogen-dependent)
estrogen dominance, 178: signs of, 179
estrogen herbs, 159
estrogen pollution, 178, 180
estrogen/progestin side effects, OCs, 191–194
estrogen replacement therapy, 5, 205 (*See also* hormone replacement therapy)
evening primrose oil, 167–168
exercise, 20, 72–73, 80, 118, 148–152, 158, 174

F
facial hair, unwanted, 190, 193, 194
fake-fat diet, 125
fallopian tubes, 22, 180
family counselor, 52
family practitioner, 100
fat, stored as glucose, 129
fat cells, 75, 76, 178
fat, desire to be, 144 (*See also* overeaters)

fat substitutes, 124–125
fats, 119,121
fatigue: chronic, 78–82; normal, 76–78
fees: alternative healing systems, 106; health care providers, ethical issue, 115; therapists, 52
Feldenkrais, Moshe, 174
Feldenkrais method, 174
female athletes, 17, 18
female doctors, 94, 108–110 (*See also* women's health movement)
feminine deodorant products, 30–31
feminine persona, 55
feminism, 8–9, 97
feminist therapy, 53, 54–56, 108
fen/phen, 5, 188
fertility drugs, 5, 42, 188
fertilized egg, 14–15
fetus, 13, 188
fiber, 119, 122, 133: fiber/water recipe, 134
fibroids, 19, 22, 25, 98, 180
fibromyalgia, 78, 80, 81
fibrositis, 78
fight or flight response, 63
first wave feminism, 8
Fitzgerald, William, 106
folate (folic acid), 128, 139
follicle-stimulating hormone (FSH), 14, 196
food addiction, 144–147
food chain, cleaning up, 181
food chemicals, 164–165
food cravings, xi, 6, 83, 122, 170, 171; sugar, 62, 83, 122
Food and Drug Administration (FDA), 28, 29,124
food, safe, 181
foods: brain, 127, 128; dosha, 102; PMS irritants, 128–130; trigger, CFS, 81
For Her Own Good (Ehrenreich/English), 8
forgiveness, stress-reliever, 132
friendships, 44–45, 77
fructose, 127, 128, 129

placenta, 15

platelet disorders, 19

pleasure: hedonism, 38; loss of. *See* anhedonia

PMS: and blood sugar, 6, 82–86, 118; and calcium deficiency, 143; charting, 34, 91–92; cultural attitudes to, 2–4, 7–8; and depression, 35–48; and eating disorders, 142–147; emotional signs, 34, 37; and hormonal fluctuations, 14–15; physical signs, 62–92; positive perspective, xi, 35; psychiatric labeling of, 7–8; and stress, 6, 35, 62–65; subclassifications, 6–7; syndrome label, 5–7

PMS defense, 95

PMS irritants, foods, 128–130

PMS — treatment: alternative healing, 6, 100, 101–107; dietary modification, xi, xii, 6, 101, 118–147; endocrinological approach, 99; exercise, 148–152; gynecological approach, 98–99; hands-on healing, 171–174; herbal therapies, 156–171; homeopathy, 169–171; natural progesterone therapy, 5, 6, 176, 182–185; naturopathic approach, 101; prescription drugs, 188–208; primary care doctor approach, 100; psychiatric approach, 97–98

pneuma (life force), 171

postmenopause, 17

post-modernist feminism, 8–9

postpartum thyroid inflammation, 87

postprandial depression, 122

post-viral fatigue syndrome, 79 (*See also* chronic fatigue syndrome)

postural drainage, 174

postural re-education strategies, 174

postures, yoga, 151

potassium, 140, 196

poverty, 41

powerlessness, 43, 45, 96

prana (life force), 106, 171

pregnancy: and domestic violence, 41; and gestational diabetes, 83; loss, 42; medicalization of, 5; and menstrual cycle, 14–15; passing clots, 19; and skipped periods, 16; "stressed," 17; unwanted, 191

premenstrual depression versus depression, 6

premenstrual dysphoric disorder. *See* PDD

premenstrual signs. *See* PMS

premenstrual syndrome, label, 5

Premenstrual Syndrome, The (Dalton), 5

premenstrual tension (PMT), x

primary care doctors, 100

primary dysmenorrhea, 21

primary menorrhagia, 18

Professional Compounding Centers of America (PCCA), 183

progesterone, 2: as contraceptive, 184–185, 189; creams, 183; deficiency, 6, 178, 191; role of, 14, 20, 83, 176 (*See also* botanical progesterone; natural progesterone therapy)

progesterone/estrogen ratio, 178

progesterone herbs, 159

progesterone receptors, 2, 35, 62–63, 82, 86, 95, 118, 135, 156, 177–178

progestin, 25, 82, 95, 177, 189, 190, 194

progestin-only Pill (POP), 191

progestin-related side effects, OCs, 193

prolactin, 76, 196

proliferatory phase, menstrual cycle, 14

prostaglandins, 23, 160, 168: drugs that inhibit, 197

Protein Power, 121

proteins, 119, 122

Prozac, x–xi, 9, 200–201

psychiatric treatment (women), social history, 7–8, 96–97

psychiatrists, 50, 52, 95–98; feminist critics of, 97

psychoanalysis, 58

psychoanalytic therapy, 58

psychodynamic therapy, 57

psychological associate, 50–51

psychologists, 50–51
psychostimulants, 205
psychotherapy, 50, 52, 57–58, 97
psycho-spiritual stress, 67
purging. *See* bulimia nervosa; chronic
    self-induced vomiting; eating disorders
Pyridoxine (Vitamin B6), 139

Q

qi (life force), 102, 103, 105, 106, 152, 171
Qi Gong exercises, 152
quitting smoking, 74–75, 130–131

R

rapid eye movement sleep (REM), 76
reabsorption time, 200
Recommended Daily Allowance, 124
Recommended Nutrient Intake (RNI), 124
rectal health, 22, 32
reflexology, 105–106, 171–172
relaxation training, 105
respect for persons. *See* patient autonomy
reversible inhibitors of monoamine oxidase
    A (RIMAs), 203
rheumatism, 78
rheumatoid arthritis, 80
riboflavin (vitamin B2), 138
Royal College of Physicians & Surgeons, 50,
    110, 115

S

saccharin, 125
St. John's wort, 82, 161–163
Salpetriere (asylum), 96
salt intake, recommendations, 129–130
SAM-e, 163
Sarafem, x, 7, 200
Schlesinger, Dr. Laura, 49–50
seasonal affective disorder (SAD), 46–48, 57,
    122
second wave feminism, 8–9
secondary dysmenorrhea, 21
secondary menorrhagia, 18

secretory phase, menstrual cycle, 14
selective serotonin reuptake inhibitors
    (SSRIs), 200, 201, 202, 203–204
selenium, 141
self-esteem, 36, 43, 46, 55, 56, 201
self, silencing, 46
self-harm, manifestation of anger, 45
self-help programs, 108, 146–147
self-massage, pressure points, 172–173
self-statements, 46
semen quality, 180
serenity prayer, 132, 146
serotonin, 6, 47, 127, 200, 201, 203
serotonin-norepinephrine reuptake
    inhibitors, 203 (*See also* selective
    serotonin reuptake inhibitors)
serving sizes, food labels, 124
sexism, 8, 12, 41, 43, 46, 97, 110 (*See also*
    feminism; patriarchy; social history,
    women)
sexual harassment, 41
sexual intercourse: during period, 12; pain
    during/after, 22, 23 (*See also* libido;
    orgasm)
sexually transmitted diseases (STDs), 20
Shamanism, 3
shame, menstruation, 4
shiatsu, 105
sialadenosis, 144
Silent Spring (Carson), 55
silicon, 141
simple carbohydrates, 118, 119, 122
simple sugars, 85, 122, 129
situational depression: causes, 39–45; signs,
    37–39; triggers, 36
sleep, 38, 47, 71, 76 (*See also* insomnia)
smoking, 25, 62, 73–74: quitting, 130–131
social history, women: psychiatry, 7–8,
    95–97; medical research, 188
social network, expanding, tips, 44–45
social workers, 51, 52
solitude versus loneliness, 44
sodium, 128, 129–130

U.S. Dept. of Health and Human Services, 188

U.S. National Institute of Health (NIH), 102: Office of Women's Health, 4

U.S. National Institute of Mental Health, 7, 163

uterus, 14, 20, 24, 99

V

vagina, 13, 22, 24: mucus, 15, 29; odor, 31–32

Vagina Monologues, The (Ensler), 4

violence, 6, 40–41, 45, 65

vitamins/minerals, 134–142

voluntariness, informed consent, 112

volunteering, 45

vomiting, chronic self-induced, 144

von Peczely, Ignatz, 104

von Willebrand's disease, 19

vulva, 22

W

water consumption, 128, 134, 144

water retention, 7, 137 (*See also* bloating)

weight gain: alcohol consumption, 71–72; and depression, 39; and eating disorders, 142, 144; feature, PMS/PDD, 7, 75; OC-related, 193; and SAD, 46; and Type 2 diabetes, 83

weight loss: and depression, 38–39; sudden, 17

well woman clinics, 108

wines, 71–72

Winfrey, Oprah, 152–153

witches, women healers, 109

women-centered medicine, 108–110

women-centered therapy. *See* feminist therapy

Women and Madness (Chesler), 8, 96

women's community centers, 110

Women's Counselling, Referral and Education Centre (Toronto), 108

women's health movement, 107–110

women's movement, 8–9 (*See also* feminism)

women's physicians, 94

workaholics, 66

workplace: stress/harassment, 41, 64; therapists, 48; toxins, 81; violence, 65

World Health Organization, 2, 29

X

xenoestrogens. *See* environmental estrogens

xylitol, 125, 127

Y

Yellow Emperor's Classic of Internal Medicine, The, 105

yin and yang, 103

ylang-ylang, 32, 165

yoga, 102, 148, 149–151

Z

zinc, 114

Zoloft, 201